THE JEMS
EMT-B CERTIFICATION PREPARATION AND REVIEW

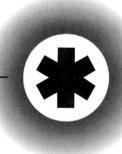

THE JEMS
EMT-B CERTIFICATION PREPARATION
AND REVIEW

DANIEL MACK, NREMT-P

President
Alternative Medical Education Concepts, Inc.
Cincinnati, Ohio

A JEMS BOOK

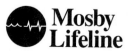

St. Louis Baltimore Boston Carlsbad Chicago Naples New York Philadelphia Portland
London Madrid Mexico City Singapore Sydney Tokyo Toronto Wiesbaden

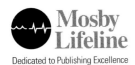

Dedicated to Publishing Excellence

A Times Mirror
Company

Publisher: David Dusthimer
Executive Editor: Claire Merrick
Acquisitions Editor: Rina Steinhauer
Assistant Editor: John Goucher
Project Manager: Chris Baumle
Production Editor: David Orzechowski
Assistant Production Editor: Susie Coladonato
Design Manager: Nancy McDonald
Manufacturing Manager: David Graybill

Printed in the United States of America
Composition by WC Brown
Printing and Binding by Maple Vail

Mosby–Year Book, Inc.
11830 Westline Industrial Drive
St. Louis, Missouri 63146

Library of Congress Cataloging-in-Publication Data
Mack, Daniel, 1960-
     The JEMS EMT-B certification preparation and review / Daniel Mack.
     p.   cm.
     ISBN 0-8151-6204-9
     1. Emergency medicine–Examinations, questions, etc. I. Journal of
emergency medical services. II. Title.
     [DNLM: 1. Emergency Medical Services–United States–examination
questions. 2. Emergencies–examination questions. WX 18.2 M153j
1996]
RC86.9.M34 1996
616.02′5′076—dc20
DNLM/DLC
for Library of Congress   95-23166
                                                CIP

97 98 99 00 1 / 9 8 7 6 5 4 3

Dedicated to Cynthia, Charles,
Betty, Tom, Mary,
and the personnel of the Miami Township Fire
and Emergency Medical Service

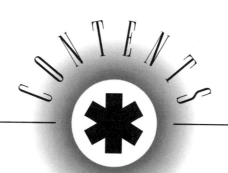

CONTENTS

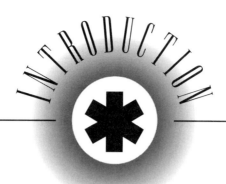

Using This Review Manual

The questions in this manual appear primarily in a multiple-choice format. This type of question not only tests knowledge of the correct answer, but also the ability to understand why an answer is incorrect. Other formats, such as matching and fill-in-the-blank are also used in this manual. These types of questions accomplish two things. First, they allow the reviewer to perform different question analysis functions. In the field, the EMT must analyze information in a variety of ways; the answer isn't there to choose from a list. Second, the use of different question formats breaks the monotony of nothing but multiple-choice questions. Keep in mind, however, that the National Registry test and certain other state tests contain only multiple-choice questions.

This review manual is not meant to take the place of a textbook or EMT instructor. Nor is it intended to simulate an actual test. There are key differences between a review manual and a test - each serves a different purpose. Due to the limited amount of space on an EMT test, there are relatively few questions in comparison with the amount of information presented in the EMT course. The test cannot be all encompassing.

✴ Enrichment Questions

This manual includes enrichment questions that cover information that may or may not have been presented in your EMT class. These are clearly identified by a "star of life" icon preceding the question number. Your exam may not contain questions covering this information. However, knowing this information may prove helpful when taking the exam and when working in the field. It can provide you with a better understanding of why patients with medical problems present in a particular way, or why certain care works best. This can increase your confidence and your abilities as an EMT.

Many tests are computer generated; questions are chosen randomly from a large bank of test questions. There is no way for the student to know exactly what will be covered. On the other hand, a review manual presents the opportunity for all or most of the critical items presented in the EMT curriculum to be covered. This allows the EMT to review specific areas of the material or, if questions are chosen randomly, a variety of information.

Getting the Most From Practice Questions

Questions on specific subjects are grouped together, allowing the EMT or student to focus on specific problem areas. This will also help the reader identify areas where additional study is needed. As you read each question, see if you can answer it without looking at the answer choices. If you answer correctly, read the rationale for the answer anyway. There may be additional helpful information included in the answer rationale.

If you answer a question incorrectly, look for a pattern. Try to determine why your answer was incorrect:

Is there a particular subject area you are having difficulty with? Or, is the missed question isolated?

If you are having difficulty with a particular subject area, concentrate on studying this section of your EMT text.

Did you not know or did you forget the information being tested? Were you unfamiliar with the subject content?

Spend extra time reviewing this material. If your time is limited, do not waste valuable study time reviewing information you already know. Concentrate on the parts of the EMT text that cover the topics you feel the least familiar with. Look for key points and definitions. Try to remember concepts, not rote answers.

Did you misunderstand the content or concept when reading the EMT text or covering the material in class? Or, did you draw a wrong conclusion when studying the topic?

Talk with your instructor or a knowledgeable EMT. Try to explain the subject using your own words and ask them what part of your explanation is incorrect. Ask for help in adjusting any misunderstanding. And don't be afraid to consult other EMT texts to compare the information presented. Each EMT text has its strong points. You may find that a different textbook presents clearer, easier to understand information on the particular subject.

Did you actually know the correct answer, but simply misread the question or answer choices?

It may be that you need to take more time to carefully read the question and answer choices. Recognizing that you have difficulty reading and comprehending test questions may be as important as identifying where additional study of the EMT materials is needed.

Did you read too much into the question?

The only information you are expected to consider is the information presented in the question stem. Do not try to determine what happened before or what might happen after the fictional "event" the question refers to.

Were you overconfident?

A positive attitude is good, but overconfidence can cause even the most competent EMT to fail.

Helpful Tips For Surviving EMT Tests

Very few people enjoy taking tests. Test taking can be even more stressful for EMT students taking an initial certification test, or for certified EMTs taking a recertification test.

Most of us got into this field because of a desire to be an EMT. It was or is a personal goal we wanted to meet. For many EMTs and EMT students, some time has elapsed since high school or college. When we were in school, the daily expectation of tests or quizzes kept us in a "test taking" frame of mind. Likely, it has been quite a while since we had to take such a critical test. And to make matters worse, we find ourselves faced with a test that will decide the course of our EMS career path.

But remember, you've come this far and you *can* pass the test. Although you may never enjoy test taking, it can be less stressful if you follow some simple, helpful hints. The more relaxed you are, the more clearly you will think. Those who write the test do not want you to fail, but they do want you to be challenged. Keeping a level head and using your sense of reasoning and problem solving will allow you to meet that challenge.

Before The Test

- Schedule time for both personal and group study. Each has its advantages. When you study alone, you have a chance to go over material you are personally unsure of. When you study in a group, you can learn from your partners and help others.

- Get plenty of rest. It's hard to think clearly if you're tired.

- Dress comfortably.

- Avoid overeating or eating foods that may be hard to digest, such as spicy or greasy foods.

Instead, eat low-fat or complex carbohydrate foods, such as nuts, pasta, or yogurt. If your test is in the morning, eat breakfast (if this is what you normally do).

- Avoid too much caffeine, which can affect attention and concentration. Do not drink alcohol prior to the test.

- Although you may feel that cramming for the test the night before will help, in general this is not the case. Cramming tends to clutter the mind and confuse the test taker.

- Give yourself enough time to reach the test location and try to arrive early. Running late for a test will only increase your anxiety. Also, by arriving early, you will have an opportunity to choose your seat wisely. Although this may not seem important, a seat in an area that is too hot, too cold, too noisy, or uncomfortable for any other reason can cause additional anxiety.

- Try to relax. If you have some favorite relaxation techniques, use them prior to starting the test. Relaxation and stress reduction exercises can also be practiced during the test provided they do not disrupt the other students. A simple exercise is to sit up straight and close your eyes. Take five deep breaths, counting each one and exhaling completely each time. As you count each breath, focus on relaxing all the muscles in your body.

- Have confidence in your ability to pass the test. Maintain a positive "I-can-pass-this-test" attitude. Put forth your best effort. Imagine how good you'll feel when you receive word that you have passed.

Tips For Multiple-Choice Test Taking

- Carefully read all the directions prior to starting the test to be sure you understand what you are supposed to do. If you don't understand test instructions, ask the test proctor for clarification.

- Carefully read the entire question before attempting to answer it. Important background information is often contained in the sentences leading up to the actual question. You don't want to lose any points because you have misread a question.

- After reading the entire question, try to answer it without looking at the choices.

Then look at the choices to see if your answer is the same as, or close to, one of the choices.

- Read all of the choices. Even if the first choice seems to be the correct answer, read the other choices so you do not overlook a better choice.

- Give all the words in the question and the answer choices equal attention. A missed or misread word can mean the difference between a correct answer and an incorrect answer.

- In most cases, assuring scene safety, ensuring an open airway, and correcting life-threatening problems take precedence. Look for answers that deal with these aspects of patient management.

- If you are unsure of an answer, leave the corresponding number on the answer sheet blank and proceed to the next question. Be careful not to get answer numbers out of sequence. Don't forget to go back to unanswered questions after completing the exam.

- Don't take a question personally. Don't get upset over a question or answer choice you don't like. This will only increase your anxiety and tension.

- Be sure the number on the answer sheet corresponds to the number of the question. Check periodically to make sure the question and answer numbering correspond.

- It is usually best to trust your first answer choice. Only change an answer if you feel you must.

- If time permits or if you are having difficulty deciding on an answer, read the question using each of the answer choices given. Reading the question and each answer choice together in their entirety allows you to focus on choices that make sense both logically and grammatically.

- The answers to multiple-choice questions do not follow a pattern, so don't try to find one. Trying to find a pattern will only add to any confusion you may already feel.

- If you do not immediately recognize the correct answer, eliminate any choice that you are sure is incorrect, so you have fewer answers to choose from. If you can narrow the number of choices to two plausible answers, you have greatly increased your chances of getting the answer right.

- Look for absolutes, such as "never," "always," or "every." These types of words may indicate that the choice is wrong.

- Look for key words in the question such as "immediately," "initially," "first," or "most." These may help you identify which answer choice is the best.

- Carefully read any question using the words "not" or "except." These types of questions are used to determine if you can tell what should not be done or if you know an exception. Many tests try to avoid such questions, but some still use them.

- Be wary of any distractors that contain words or information you have never seen, even if they seem to be plausible choices.

- Base your answers on what you learned from the text, not an experience other practicing EMTs may have had with different patients.

- If you are allowed to use a sheet of paper to solve problems, take advantage of it.

Managing Your Time

- Know how much time is allotted for the test and how many questions you must answer. For instance, the National Registry test allows 2 hours and 30 minutes to complete 150 questions (which averages out to 1 minute per question). In most cases, you will be given more time than you are likely to need. Relax and do not be overly time conscious early on.

- Use all the allotted time. Only knowledge is being tested, not your ability to finish early.

- When taking the exam, try to answer the easiest questions first. Save the harder questions for last. Doing so will allow you to spend more time on the harder questions.

- Make sure you go back to all the questions you have left blank. If unanswered questions count against you, take a guess if you still don't know the answer.

- If you have time left at the end of the exam, review your answers. Sometimes the content of a later question or answer may remind you of information that could affect a previous answer.

- Check your answer sheet. Be sure each choice marked on the answer sheet corresponds to the choice you want. Even if you know the answer to a question, marking errors can cause the choice to be scored as incorrect. Also check to be sure you did not leave any questions unanswered.

A word of caution applies when using this or any review manual. Do not view this book as a review manual to pass the National Registry test or any other particular test. If you are taking the National Registry test, some questions may be presented differently. Do not become overly confident simply because you have completed a review manual. Passing tests does not make you a good EMT. Instead, if you try to be the most knowledgeable and best EMT you can be, passing the test will be an added bonus. We wish you the best in your endeavors to become, or remain, the best EMT you can be.

NOTE TO THE READER: The Author and publisher have made every attempt to assure that the drug dosages and patient care procedures presented in this text are accurate and represent accepted practices in the United States. They are not provided as standards of care. It is the reader's responsibility to follow patient care protocols established by medical direction physicians and to remain current in the delivery of emergency care.

CHAPTER 1

THE HUMAN BODY

THE SKELETAL SYSTEM

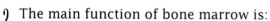

1. The functions of the skeletal system include:
   a. protecting vital organs
   b. providing form
   c. providing for body movement
   d. all of the above

✱ 2. The main function of bone marrow is:
   a. regulation of body temperature
   b. production of insulin
   c. production of red blood cells
   d. regulation of body metabolism

3. Using the following list, label Figure 1-1.
   mandible, maxilla, nasal bone, orbit, zygomatic bone

4. The largest bone of the pelvis is the:
   a. ischium
   b. ilium
   c. pubis
   d. acetabulum

5. The rib cage is comprised of:
   a. 12 pairs of ribs, all attached to the sternum
   b. 10 pairs of ribs, eight attached to the sternum and two floating
   c. 10 pairs of ribs, all attached to the sternum
   d. 12 pairs of ribs, 10 attached to the sternum and two floating

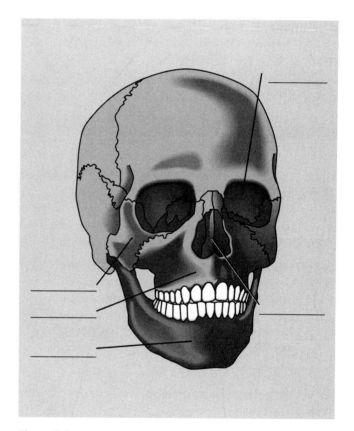

Figure 1-1

✱ 6. The lower, movable section of the jaw is the:
   a. maxilla
   b. mastoid
   c. mandible
   d. malleolus

7. The upper segment of the sternum is the:
   a. flagellum
   b. angle of Louis
   c. manubrium
   d. anacronym

8. The small, finger-like projection of cartilage at the inferior end of the sternum is the:
   a. mastoid process
   b. xiphoid process
   c. styloid process
   d. lenticular process

9. The heel bone is also known as the:
   a. calcaneus
   b. metacarpals
   c. carpals
   d. metatarsals

10. The greater trochanter is part of the:
    a. radius
    b. lumbar spine
    c. tibia
    d. femur

11. The kneecap is also called the:
    a. parietal
    b. peronia
    c. planum
    d. patella

12. Using the given list of sections of the spine, label Figure 1-2.
    cervical, coccyx, lumbar, thoracic, sacrum

13. The collar bone is the:
    a. scapula
    b. clavicle
    c. acromion process
    d. costal cartilage

14. Referring to Figure 1-3, use the list of bones below to label the upper and lower extremities.
    carpals, clavicle, femur, fibula, humerus, metacarpals, metatarsals, patella, phalanges, radius, tarsals, tibia, ulna

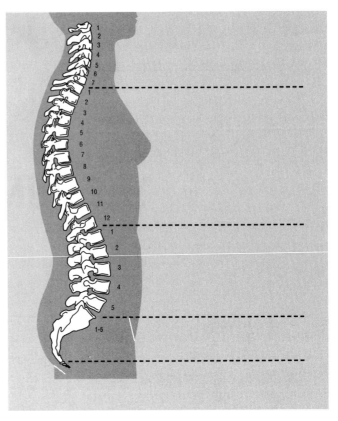

Figure 1-2

 15. Three bones lying directly underneath the skin that can be palpated throughout their entire length are the:
    a. femur, tibia, and fibula
    b. humerus, radius, and ulna
    c. tibia, clavicle, and ulna
    d. femur, clavicle, and humerus

16. An example of a ball-and-socket joint is the:
    a. elbow
    b. finger
    c. metatarsals
    d. hip

17. The knee joint is an example of a:
    a. hinge joint
    b. ball-and-socket joint
    c. floating joint
    d. false joint

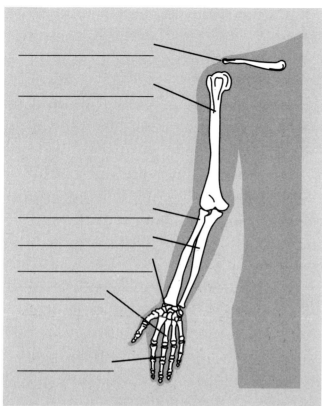

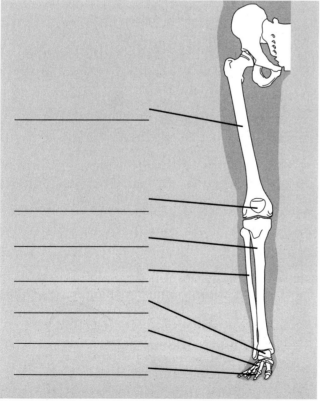

Figure 1-3 Upper extremities, *top*
Lower extremities, *bottom*

THE MUSCULAR SYSTEM

✱ 18. Concerning the function of muscles, a true statement is:
   a. muscles don't pull, only push
   b. muscles don't push, only pull
   c. muscles both push and pull
   d. none of the above

19. The type of muscle found in the gastrointestinal tract is:
   a. skeletal
   b. cardiac
   c. smooth
   d. striated

20. The type of muscle that allows you to move an arm or a leg is:
   a. skeletal
   b. smooth
   c. cardiac
   d. involuntary

✱ 21. The diaphragm differs from most skeletal muscles in that it:
   a. primarily acts as an involuntary muscle
   b. is not striated
   c. is formed from smooth muscle
   d. is formed from cardiac muscle

22. The ability of cardiac muscle to contract on its own is known as:
   a. self-regulation
   b. focality
   c. external pacing
   d. automaticity

THE SKIN

23. Two main functions of the skin are:
   a. blood cell production and waste disposal
   b. temperature regulation and fluid absorption
   c. protection and temperature regulation
   d. waste disposal and fluid absorption

24. The outermost layer of the skin is known as the:
   a. epidermis
   b. superdermis
   c. subcutaneous layer
   d. hyperdermis

25. The sweat glands and hair follicles are contained in the:
   a. dermis
   b. subcutaneous layer
   c. fascia
   d. subarachnoid layer

 26. Sebaceous glands secrete:
   a. acids
   b. sweat
   c. saliva
   d. oils

27. Directly beneath the dermis lies the:
   a. bone
   b. subcutaneous layer
   c. meninges
   d. subfascia layer

THE NERVOUS SYSTEM

28. The two anatomical divisions of the nervous system are the:
   a. central nervous system and peripheral nervous system
   b. automatic nervous system and somatic nervous system
   c. central nervous system and automatic nervous system
   d. peripheral nervous system and systemic nervous system

29. The central nervous system consists of the:
   a. brain and spinal cord
   b. nervous and integumentary systems
   c. automatic nervous system and spinal cord
   d. brain and cranial nerves

30. The two main types of nerves that enter and leave the spinal cord are:
   a. neuron and proton
   b. peripheral and motor
   c. lateral and medial
   d. sensory and motor

31. Higher functions, such as thought, decision making, and communication are the responsibility of the:
   a. autonomic nervous system
   b. somatic nervous system
   c. central nervous system
   d. cranial nervous system

THE RESPIRATORY SYSTEM

32. The structure that prevents food or liquids from entering the trachea is the:
   a. uvula
   b. epinephrine
   c. cardiac sphincter
   d. epiglottis

33. Tidal volume refers to the:
   a. volume of blood passing through the lungs
   b. regularity of breathing
   c. volume of air per breath
   d. rate of breathing

34. The two gases normally exchanged during breathing are:
   a. oxygen and carbon monoxide
   b. nitrogen and oxygen
   c. carbon dioxide and nitrogen
   d. oxygen and carbon dioxide

35. The structure commonly referred to as the "Adam's apple" is the:
   a. cricothyroid membrane
   b. thyroid cartilage
   c. sixth tracheal ring
   d. esophageal sphincter

36. The major muscle associated with breathing mechanics is the:
    a. quadricep
    b. deltoid
    c. pectoral
    d. diaphragm

✳ 37. The primary stimulus for breathing in normal, healthy humans is the:
    a. oxygen level in arterial blood
    b. carbon monoxide level in venous blood
    c. carbon dioxide level in arterial blood
    d. oxygen level in venous blood

38. The exchange of gases within the lungs takes place in the:
    a. bronchi
    b. pleural space
    c. alveoli
    d. trachea

39. When blood enters the capillaries in the lungs, it is:
    a. high in oxygen and low in carbon dioxide
    b. low in oxygen and high in carbon dioxide
    c. low in oxygen and low in carbon dioxide
    d. high in oxygen and high in carbon dioxide

40. When blood enters the capillaries at the body tissue level, it is:
    a. low in oxygen and low in carbon dioxide
    b. high in oxygen and high in carbon dioxide
    c. low in oxygen and high in carbon dioxide
    d. high in oxygen and low in carbon dioxide

THE CIRCULATORY SYSTEM

41. The chambers of the heart that receive blood are the:
    a. atria
    b. ventricles
    c. aorta
    d. vallecula

42. The chambers of the heart that pump blood are the:
    a. atria
    b. ventricles
    c. varices
    d. auricles

✳ 43. The muscular wall that separates the right and left sides of the heart is the:
    a. cardiac divisor
    b. sacrum
    c. septum
    d. diaphragm

44. The heart muscle receives oxygen and nourishment via the:
    a. coronary arteries
    b. ventricles
    c. pulmonary veins
    d. mitral valves

45. The major artery originating from the heart is the:
    a. carotid
    b. innominate
    c. aorta
    d. subclavian

✳ 46. The amount of blood in an average-sized adult is:
    a. 5 pints
    b. 5 liters
    c. 5 units
    d. 5 gallons

47. Blood is pumped to the body by the:
    a. left atrium
    b. left ventricle
    c. right auricle
    d. right varices

48. Blood is pumped to the lungs by the:
    a. left auricle
    b. left varices
    c. right atrium
    d. right ventricle

49. The average amount of blood in a 1-year-old child is:
   a. 8 pints
   b. 3 liters
   c. 800 cc
   d. 5 units

50. The functions of blood include:
   a. carrying oxygen and removing waste products
   b. combatting infections
   c. clotting capabilities
   d. all of the above

51. Mark the following list of characteristics as applying to:
   A = arteries C = capillaries V = veins
   ___ carry blood to the heart
   ___ carry blood away from the heart
   ___ have thin walls which allow exchange of oxygen and nutrients with cells
   ___ carry blood under high pressure

52. White blood cells are responsible for:
   a. carrying oxygen
   b. carrying carbon dioxide
   c. removing wastes
   d. defending against infection

53. The liquid component of blood is known as:
   a. whole blood
   b. plasma
   c. lymph
   d. melanoma

54. Red blood cells are responsible for:
   a. carrying oxygen
   b. maintaining blood acidity
   c. carrying carbon monoxide
   d. filtering blood impurities

55. The small, disc-shaped components of blood essential to the formation of blood clots are:
   a. T-cells
   b. fibrocytes
   c. electrolytes
   d. platelets

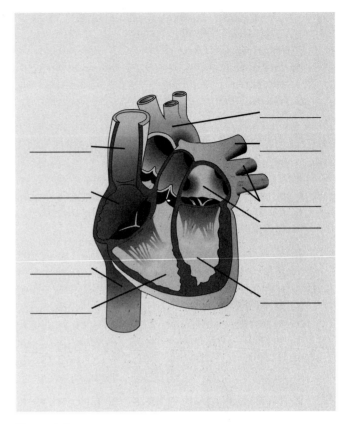

Figure 1-4

56. Using the following list of components of the circulatory system, label Figure 1-4.
   aorta, inferior vena cava, left atrium, left ventricle, pulmonary artery, pulmonary veins, right atrium, right ventricle, superior vena cava

GENERAL ANATOMY AND PHYSIOLOGY

57. The endocrine system is responsible for producing:
   a. chemicals
   b. red blood cells
   c. sugar and glucose
   d. white blood cells

58. The spine is located on the:
   a. ventral side
   b. cephalic side
   c. anterior side
   d. dorsal side

59. In anatomical terms, the umbilicus is on the:
a. anterior abdomen
b. caudal abdomen
c. posterior abdomen
d. lateral abdomen

60. A body structure that is above another is:
a. lateral
b. superior
c. distal
d. inferior

61. The fingers are on the:
a. lateral end of the arm
b. proximal end of the arm
c. distal end of the arm
d. medial end of the arm

✱ **62.** When describing something that appears or is present on both sides of the body, EMTs should use the term:
a. hemilateral
b. bilateral
c. trilateral
d. bigeminy

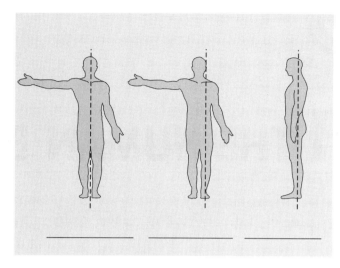

Figure 1-5

63. Using the three imaginary dividing lines, label Figure 1-5.
midaxillary line, midclavicular line, midline

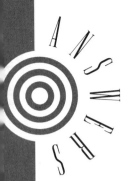

1 THE HUMAN BODY

1. **d.** All of the above. The skeletal system protects vital organs, provides form for the body, and provides for body movement. It also produces blood cells.

2. **c.** Bone marrow produces red blood cells.

3.

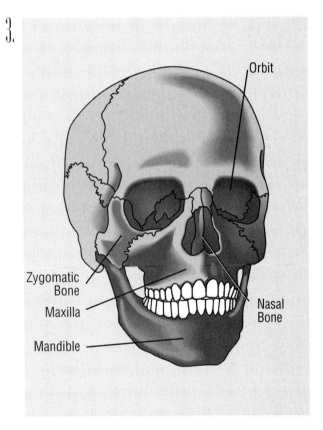

Orbit

Zygomatic Bone

Maxilla

Mandible

Nasal Bone

Figure 1-1

4. **b.** The ilium is the largest bone of the pelvis. The ischium and pubis are the other two bones of the pelvis. The acetabulum is the rounded cavity of the pelvis into which the femoral head fits.

5. **d.** The human body contains 12 pairs of ribs. Ten pairs attach to the sternum. The lower two pairs do not and are therefore "floating."

6. **c.** The mandible is the lower, movable section of the jaw. The maxilla is the upper jaw. The malleolus is the rounded projection on either side of the ankle joint.

7. **c.** The manubrium is the upper segment of the sternum. The main, middle segment of the sternum is the body. The angle of Louis is a bony prominence at the level of the second rib that marks the junction of the manubrium and body of the sternum.

8. **b.** The xiphoid process is the cartilaginous projection at the lower end of the sternum. The styloid process and mastoid process are parts of the skull. The lenticular process is part of the incus bone of the middle ear.

9. **a.** The calcaneus is the heel bone. The carpals and metacarpals are bones of the hand and wrist. The metatarsals are bones of the foot.

10. **d.** The greater trochanter is part of the femur.

11. **d.** The patella is the kneecap. Parietal pertains to the wall of a cavity.

12.

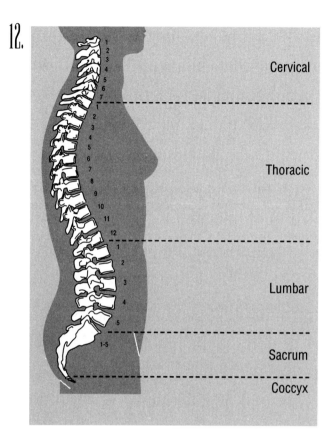

Cervical

Thoracic

Lumbar

Sacrum

Coccyx

Figure 1-2

13. **b.** The clavicle is the collar bone. The scapula is the shoulder blade. The acromion process is the highest point of the shoulder and the costal cartilage connects the ribs to the sternum.

14.

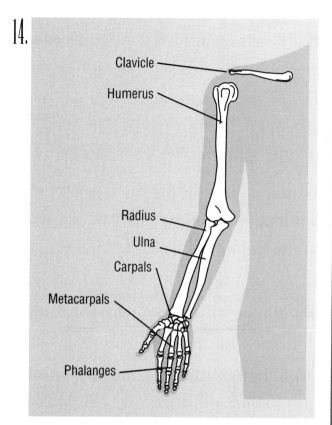

Clavicle

Humerus

Radius

Ulna

Carpals

Metacarpals

Phalanges

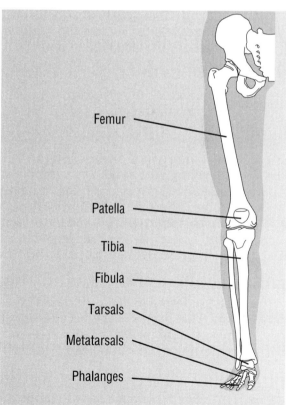

Femur

Patella

Tibia

Fibula

Tarsals

Metatarsals

Phalanges

Figure 1-3

15. **c.** The tibia, clavicle, and ulna lie directly underneath the skin and can be palpated their entire length.

16. **d.** The hip is an example of a ball-and-socket joint, as is the shoulder.

17. **a.** The knee and elbow are hinge joints. A false joint is one that forms subsequent to a broken bone.

18. **b.** Muscles DON'T push, ONLY pull.

19. **c.** The gastrointestinal tract is made up of smooth muscle. Smooth muscles are also referred to as involuntary muscles.

20. **a.** Skeletal muscles allow us to move. They are also classified as voluntary muscles.

21. **a.** The diaphragm acts primarily as an involuntary muscle even though it is formed of striated skeletal muscle.

22. **d.** Automaticity refers to cardiac muscle's ability to contract on its own.

23. **c.** The skin provides protection to underlying structures and temperature regulation. Because it is rich in nerve endings, the skin also allows information to be transmitted from the environment to the brain. The skin senses heat, cold, touch, pressure, and pain.

24. **a.** The epidermis is the outermost layer of skin. The dermis is the second layer of the skin. Epi means "upon," therefore epidermis means upon the dermis.

25. **a.** The dermis contains sweat glands and hair follicles.

26. **d.** Oils are secreted by sebaceous glands.

27. **b.** The subcutaneous layer is a layer of fatty tissue that lies under the dermis.

28. **a.** The two anatomical divisions of the nervous system are the central nervous system and peripheral nervous system.

29. **a.** The brain and spinal cord make up the central nervous system.

30. **d.** Sensory and motor nerves are the two main types of nerves that enter and leave the spinal cord.

31. **c.** The central nervous system is responsible for higher mental functions, including thought, decision making, and communication. Additionally, it plays an important role in regulating body functions.

32. **d.** The epiglottis prevents food or liquids from entering the trachea. The uvula is the structure that hangs down from the soft palate above the back of the tongue. The cardiac sphincter closes the esophageal opening of the stomach.

33. **c.** Tidal volume refers to the volume of air per breath. It is a measure of how deeply the patient is breathing.

34. **d.** Oxygen and carbon dioxide are normally exchanged during breathing.

35. **b.** The thyroid cartilage is commonly referred to as the Adam's apple. It is part of the larynx.

36. **d.** The diaphragm is the major muscle involved in breathing. It also separates the thoracic cavity from the abdominal cavity. Intercostal muscles are also involved in breathing.

37. c. In healthy humans, the carbon dioxide level in arterial blood is the most sensitive and rapidly responding system for breathing stimulus. A secondary stimulus is a low level of oxygen in arterial blood.

38. c. The exchange of gases during breathing takes place in the alveoli. The alveoli, resembling small grape clusters, are the "work stations" of the lungs.

39. b. Blood entering the capillaries in the lungs is low in oxygen and high in carbon dioxide.

40. d. Since blood reaching the body tissues has come from the lungs, it is high in oxygen and low in carbon dioxide.

41. a. The atria receive blood. They are the upper chambers of the heart. Atria is plural; the singular form is atrium. The vallecula is the depression between the epiglottis and the root of the tongue.

42. b. The ventricles pump the blood. They are the lower chambers of the heart. Varices are dilated, twisted blood vessels. The atria are sometimes referred to as the auricles.

43. c. The right and left sides of the heart are separated by a muscular wall known as the septum.

44. a. The coronary arteries supply the heart muscle with blood. Pulmonary veins carry blood from the lungs to the heart.

45. c. The aorta is the major artery in the body and comes directly off the heart. It is also the largest artery. The carotid, subclavian, and innominate (or brachiocephalic) arteries branch off the arch of the aorta.

46. b. The average-sized adult has 5 liters (approximately 10 pints) of blood. Blood volume may be less in females and smaller males. Generally, about $1/12$ to $1/15$ (or 7%) of body weight is blood.

47. b. The left ventricle pumps blood to the body. The left atrium receives blood from the lungs.

48. d. Blood is pumped to the lungs by the right ventricle. The right atrium receives blood from the body.

49. c. The average amount of blood in a 1-year-old child is approximately 800 cc.

50. d. All of the above. Blood carries oxygen, removes waste products, including carbon dioxide, carries antibodies that combat infections, and carries clotting factors.

51.
   _V_ carry blood to the heart
   _A_ carry blood away from the heart
   _C_ have thin walls which allow exchange of oxygen and nutrients with cells
   _A_ carry blood under high pressure

52. d. White blood cells defend against infection. They are also known as leukocytes (*leuko* meaning white and *cyte* meaning cell).

53. b. Plasma is the liquid component of blood. It carries the blood cells and nutrients.

54. a. Red blood cells carry oxygen. They are also known as erythrocytes (*erythro* meaning red; *cyte* meaning cell). Hemoglobin is a protein component of red blood cells that allows them to carry oxygen. Red blood cells give blood its color.

55. **d.** Platelets are small, disc-shaped components of the blood that are essential to clot formation.

56.

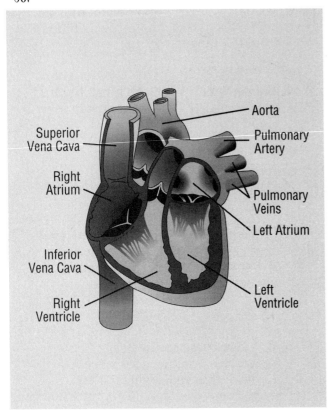

Labels: Superior Vena Cava, Right Atrium, Inferior Vena Cava, Right Ventricle, Aorta, Pulmonary Artery, Pulmonary Veins, Left Atrium, Left Ventricle

Figure 1-4

57. **a.** The endocrine system is responsible for producing chemicals that are called hormones. One hormone that is produced is insulin, which allows the body to use sugar.

58. **d.** The spine is located on the dorsal side. Ventral refers to the belly side, cephalic toward the head, and anterior is toward the front.

59. **a.** Anatomically, the umbilicus is on the anterior abdomen. Caudal is toward the tail, posterior means following or located behind, and lateral refers to away from the midline.

60. **b.** A body structure that is above another is said to be superior. Inferior refers to a structure below another.

61. **c.** The fingers are on the distal end of the arm, that is, near the end of an extremity or farther from the midline. Proximal refers to the end of an extremity closer to the midline. Medial refers to close to the midline, lateral farther from the midline.

62. **b.** The term bilateral refers to something being on both sides of the body.

63.

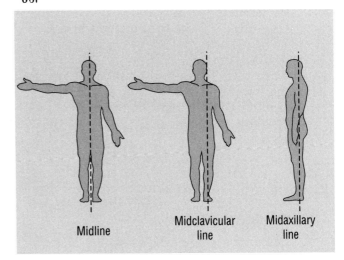

Labels: Midline, Midclavicular line, Midaxillary line

Figure 1-5

VITAL SIGNS AND PATIENT HISTORY

1. The chief complaint is a:
   a. list of what is currently wrong with the patient
   b. brief one-word or short description of why EMS was called
   c. history of the present illness
   d. problem with the director of an EMS

2. When assessing a child, the most important aspect is the:
   a. patient's blood pressure
   b. patient's pulse rate
   c. parent's general reactions
   d. EMT's general impression of the patient

3. Baseline vital signs consist of assessing:
   a. pulse, breathing, blood pressure, skin, and pupils
   b. breathing, pulse, medical history, and age
   c. age, sex, blood pressure, and pulse
   d. pulse, breathing, skin, and race

 4. When using a stethoscope, the earpieces should:
   a. face backward
   b. be placed in the most comfortable position
   c. face away from the patient
   d. face forward

5. The diaphragm of the stethoscope is best used for listening to:
   a. high-frequency sounds
   b. low-frequency sounds
   c. heart sounds
   d. gallops

6. When assessing breathing:
   a. instruct the patient to breath in a normal, relaxed manner
   b. place the patient in a sitting position
   c. do not let the patient know you are counting breaths
   d. ask the patient about their chief complaint and medical history

7. The normal adult breathing rate is:
   a. 5–10 breaths per minute
   b. 8–16 breaths per minute
   c. 12–20 breaths per minute
   d. 16–28 breaths per minute

8. The normal breathing rate of children is:
   a. 10–20 breaths per minute
   b. 15–30 breaths per minute
   c. 25–40 breaths per minute
   d. slower than the normal adult rate

9. The normal breathing rate of infants is:
   a. slower than the normal adult rate
   b. 10–25 breaths per minute
   c. 20–40 breaths per minute
   d. 25–50 breaths per minute

10. The EMT should be concerned if an adult has a breathing rate of:
   a. <6 or >12
   b. <8 or >24
   c. <8 or >18
   d. <14 or >20

11. Breathing characterized by occasional, gasping breaths is known as:
   a. Kussmaul breathing
   b. agonal breathing
   c. grunting breathing
   d. sonorous breathing

12. The pulse may be defined as:
   a. the number of times the heart contracts each minute
   b. the pressure in an artery
   c. a wave of blood that courses through an artery as the heart contracts
   d. blood flowing through a vein

13. When checking a carotid pulse, the EMT should:
   a. check only one side at a time
   b. check both sides simultaneously
   c. only perform carotid pulse checks on patients older than 65 years
   d. use the thumb of the hand closest to the patient's head

14. The most common place to check a pulse is the:
   a. brachial artery
   b. radial artery
   c. carotid artery
   d. femoral artery

15. The normal pulse range for an adult is:
   a. 50–70 beats per minute
   b. 60–100 beats per minute
   c. 80–120 beats per minute
   d. >110 beats per minute

16. The normal pulse range for a child is:
   a. 60–80 beats per minute
   b. 80–100 beats per minute
   c. <80 beats per minute
   d. >120 beats per minute

17. The EMT should check a pulse for:
   a. rate and quality
   b. volume and strength
   c. flow and rate
   d. quality and volume

18. The pulse rate for an infant is normally:
   a. 50–80 beats per minute
   b. 80–100 beats per minute
   c. 100–140 beats per minute
   d. 170–200 beats per minute

19. To quickly assess a patient's skin temperature:
   a. touch the patient's skin with the back of the hand
   b. touch the patient's skin with the palm of the hand
   c. kiss the patient's forehead
   d. touch the patient's lips with the back of the hand

20. Capillary refill time should be checked:
   a. on patients older than 16 years
   b. on all patients
   c. on any patient in shock
   d. on patients younger than 6 years

21. When checking capillary refill time, color should normally return within:
   a. ½–1 second
   b. 2 seconds
   c. 4 seconds
   d. 10 seconds

22. For the following list of medical emergencies, note whether you would expect the patient's skin color to be: **cyanotic, flushed, jaundiced, pale, or pink**
   _____ hypoglycemia
   _____ heat emergency with dry skin
   _____ liver dysfunction
   _____ normal skin
   _____ carbon monoxide poisoning
   _____ insufficient circulation
   _____ inadequate oxygenation
   _____ hypoperfusion

23. The best place to check for jaundice is:
a. the white area of the eye
b. the lowest areas of the body
c. the gums
d. the skin of the thigh

24. Skin color may be most easily assessed by checking any of the following areas *except* the:
a. conjunctiva
b. oral mucosa
c. nail beds
d. chest

25. The skin of a patient who is in hypoperfusion (shock) is most likely to be:
a. flushed, cool, and dry
b. cyanotic, warm, and dry
c. flushed, warm, and moist
d. pale, cool, and moist

26. When checking pupils, the EMT should remember that:
a. cataracts do not affect pupil response
b. unequal pupils generally occur early in head injuries
c. medications may affect pupillary response
d. bright lights will not affect the pupil check

✱ 27. Normal pupils are:
a. unequal and constrict when exposed to light
b. equal and constrict when exposed to light
c. dilated and become unequal when exposed to light
d. constricted and dilate when exposed to light

28. Blood pressure can be defined as:
a. the pressure blood exerts against the walls of the arteries
b. the pulse in an artery
c. the pressure exerted by blood against the walls of the veins
d. the difference between the arterial pressure and venous pressure

29. A blood pressure should be checked on:
a. patients experiencing a rapid heart rate
b. every patient regardless of the type of incident
c. patients older than 3 years
d. only patients who have sustained trauma

✱ 30. To obtain an accurate reading, the width of the blood pressure cuff bladder should be:
a. the length of the forearm
b. at least 20% greater than the diameter of the patient's arm
c. twice the diameter of the arm
d. 60% of the limb circumference

✱ 31. An error in blood pressure measurement may be the result of:
a. incorrect cuff size
b. operator error
c. loud background noise
d. all of the above

32. The first sound noted when taking a blood pressure by auscultation is the:
a. diastolic pressure
b. systolic pressure
c. mean arterial pressure
d. venous pressure

33. The diastolic pressure corresponds to:
a. the pressure exerted against the walls of the arteries when the heart is pumping
b. the difference between the resting pressure and pumping pressure
c. the pressure exerted against the walls of the arteries when the left ventricle is at rest
d. half the systolic pressure

34. Systolic blood pressure may indicate a serious problem if it is:
a. >90 mm Hg
b. >130 mm Hg
c. <100 mm Hg
d. <140 mm Hg

35. Obtaining a blood pressure by feeling a pulse rather than by listening with a stethoscope is known as:
   a. auscultating a blood pressure
   b. palpating a blood pressure
   c. pulsing a blood pressure
   d. tamponading a blood pressure

36. If the EMT encounters difficulty hearing a blood pressure, the sounds may be augmented by:
   a. slowly inflating the cuff
   b. lowering the arm before inflating the cuff
   c. elevating the arm before inflating the cuff
   d. rapidly deflating the cuff

37. To obtain an accurate reading, a blood pressure cuff should be deflated at a rate of:
   a. 1–2 mm Hg a second
   b. 2–3 mm Hg a second
   c. 3–4 mm Hg a second
   d. 4–5 mm Hg a second

38. When charting vital signs on a run report, always note the:
   a. name of the EMT taking the vital signs
   b. arm used to take the pulse and blood pressure
   c. position the patient was in while vital signs were taken
   d. time the vital signs were taken

39. A second set of vital signs should always be checked before the patient reaches the hospital in order to:
   a. make the run report appear more complete
   b. confirm that the first set is correct
   c. compare with the initial set for changes
   d. provide the EMT with additional practice in taking vital signs

40. Vital signs on an unstable patient should be checked:
   a. every 5 minutes
   b. every 10 minutes
   c. every 15 minutes
   d. only if a medical intervention is performed

For questions 41 to 46, refer to the mnemonic S-A-M-P-L-E.

41. When the EMT takes a patient history, the letter "P" refers to:
   a. location of "pain"
   b. presence of "paralysis"
   c. events "preceding" the injury or illness
   d. "pertinent" past medical history

42. The letter "M" refers to:
   a. present "medications"
   b. ability to "move" all extremities
   c. time of the last "meal"
   d. name of the patient's "MD"

43. The letter "E" refers to:
   a. length of time from onset of problem until "EMS" was called
   b. "events" leading up to the injury or illness
   c. whether the situation should be classified as a true "emergency"
   d. whether there is a need for "extrication"

44. The letter "L" refers to:
   a. the patient's "lifestyle"
   b. things that "lead" up to the event
   c. the patient's "last" oral intake
   d. checking the patient's "lung" sounds

45. When routinely questioning a patient about allergies (the "A" in S-A-M-P-L-E), the EMT should be most concerned with allergies to:
a. medications
b. food
c. environmental factors
d. all of the above

46. Something related to a patient's medical problem that the EMT sees, feels, or hears is a:
a. symptom
b. syndrome
c. sign
d. scenario

47. From the following list, mark whether each is a:

sign, symptom, or both

_____ chest pain
_____ cyanosis
_____ apnea
_____ difficulty breathing
_____ nausea
_____ sweating
_____ cool skin
_____ headache
_____ dizziness
_____ paleness
_____ deformed extremity
_____ vomiting
_____ swelling
_____ double vision
_____ numbness
_____ wheezing

ADDITIONAL POINTS FOR DISCUSSION

1. The medications taken by a patient can give the EMT a clue regarding what kind of medical problems a patient has. Because many patients are poor historians (especially the elderly), it is good for the EMT to be familiar with prescription medications commonly taken for certain medical problems. Review previous emergency calls to which you have responded. What medications are most commonly associated with the following problems:

* Heart problems:

* Breathing problems:

* High blood pressure (hypertension):

* Diabetes:

* Seizure disorders:

* Abdominal disorders:

* Behavioral problems:

2. Research some of the medications you have listed in a drug reference book and become familiar with their actions and side effects.

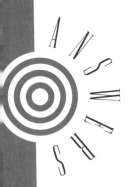

2 VITAL SIGNS AND PATIENT HISTORY

1. **b.** The chief complaint is a brief one-word or short description of why EMS was called.

2. **d.** The EMT's general impression of a sick or injured child is more important than vital signs. Children can maintain what appear to be normal vital signs but their condition can suddenly deteriorate.

3. **a.** Baseline vital signs consist of assessing the pulse, breathing, blood pressure, skin, and pupils.

4. **d.** The earpieces of a stethoscope should face forward to match the natural direction of the EMT's ear canals.

5. **a.** The diaphragm of the stethoscope best amplifies high-frequency sounds, such as breath sounds. The bell is used to listen to low-frequency sounds, such as heart sounds. Gallops are types of heart sounds.

6. **c.** When assessing breathing, do not let the patient know you are counting breaths as this can affect the way the patient breathes. The patient does not need to be sitting up and should not talk during the assessment.

7. **c.** The normal adult breathing rate is 12–20 breaths per minute.

8. **b.** The normal breathing rate for children is 15–30 breaths per minute.

9. **d.** Infants may breathe 25–50 times a minute. The rate is faster than the adult rate because of an infant's rapid metabolism.

10. **b.** If the breathing rate falls below eight breaths a minute in an adult, the EMT should be concerned. Rapid breathing rates may also provide cause for alarm. Sustained rates of 24 or more breaths a minute may result in insufficient air volume. Sustained rates of greater than 28 breaths a minute are especially dangerous. Some people, such as athletes, may normally breathe slower. Always consider how the patient's problem and overall condition relate to the breathing rate and care for the patient accordingly.

11. **b.** Agonal breathing is characterized by occasional, gasping breaths and most commonly occurs immediately before death.

12. c. The pulse may be defined as a wave of blood that courses through an artery as the heart contracts. It is not the number of times the heart contracts each minute. There are times, such as when a patient has a rapid heart rate, that the heart may not completely refill. It does contract, but no pulse can be felt as there is not enough blood in the ventricles to push.

13. a. When checking a carotid pulse, check only one side at a time. Checking both sides simultaneously may obstruct blood flow to the brain. Rubbing the carotid artery may cause a drop in pulse rate, especially in the elderly. Never use the thumb to check any pulses; it has its own pulse.

14. b. EMTs most commonly check the radial pulse in any patient older than 1 year. If the radial pulse cannot be felt, assess the carotid pulse. For children younger than 1 year, check the brachial pulse.

15. b. The normal adult pulse range is 60–100 beats per minute. Remember that the overall patient picture is more important than focusing on the patient's exact pulse rate.

16. b. The normal pulse range for a child is 80–100 beats per minute. In younger children, the pulse rate may normally be greater than 100.

17. a. The pulse should be checked for rate and quality. Quality refers to volume (strong or weak) and regularity. If it is irregular, check for a regular irregularity (i.e., an extra beat every second or third beat) or irregular irregularity (i.e., no pattern to the irregularity).

18. c. The pulse rate of an infant is normally 100–140 beats per minute. The pulse rate of a newborn may be as high as 150–160.

19. a. A patient's temperature can most easily be felt with the back of the EMT's hand. Exact temperature is not as important as noting the presence of a possible fever or possible hypothermia. Lip contact should be avoided to preclude possible infection transmission.

20. d. Capillary refill time should only be checked on patients younger than 6 years. Remember that if the patient's extremities are cold, capillary refill time will not be an accurate indicator.

21. b. When checking capillary refill, the color should return within 2 seconds.

22.

pale	hypoglycemia
flushed	heat emergency with dry skin
jaundiced	liver dysfunction
pink	normal skin
flushed	carbon monoxide poisoning
pale	insufficient circulation
cyanotic	inadequate oxygenation
pale	hypoperfusion

23. a. Jaundice manifests early in the white area of the eye. This area is easy to see, and no clothing must be removed to view it.

24. d. The chest is not a good area to check for abnormal skin color. The EMT can examine the patient's conjunctiva (eyes), oral mucosa (gums and lips), or nail beds.

25. d. The skin of a patient in hypoperfusion (shock) is most likely to be pale, cool, and moist.

26. c. Medications and cataracts may affect pupillary response. Although unequal pupils may be seen in head injuries, they are usually a late sign. The EMT must also remember that many people have normally unequal pupils. Always check pupils in subdued light.

27. **b.** Normal pupils are equal and constrict when exposed to light.

28. **a.** Blood pressure is the pressure that blood exerts against the walls of the arteries.

29. **c.** Blood pressure should be checked on all patients older than 3 years.

30. **b.** The width of the blood pressure cuff bladder should be at least 20% greater than the diameter of the patient's arm or 40% of the limb circumference.

31. **d.** All of the above. Incorrect cuff size, operator error, and loud background noise can all cause inaccurate blood pressure measurements.

32. **b.** The first sound noted when taking a blood pressure by auscultation is the systolic pressure. The point when the sounds fade or disappear during deflation of the cuff corresponds with the diastolic pressure.

33. **c.** The diastolic reading corresponds with the pressure exerted against the walls of the arteries when the left ventricle is at rest. The systolic reading is the pressure during ventricular contraction.

34. **c.** A systolic blood pressure less than 100 mm Hg may indicate a serious problem, especially if the patient has associated signs and symptoms of trauma or a medical problem.

35. **b.** Palpating a blood pressure. To do this, the EMT feels a pulse below the blood pressure cuff, then inflates the cuff. When the pulse is no longer felt, the cuff is inflated another 30 mm Hg. The pressure is then released. The first pulse felt as the cuff is deflated is the systolic pressure. Palpated blood pressures should be noted as the systolic pressure over "P" (i.e., 126/P).

36. **c.** Elevating the arm prior to inflating the cuff may reduce venous congestion, which makes it difficult to hear blood pressure sounds. The cuff should be rapidly, not slowly, inflated in 7 seconds or less. The cuff should then be deflated slowly.

37. **b.** A blood pressure cuff should be deflated at a rate of 2–3 mm Hg a second.

38. **d.** EMTs should always note the time vital signs were taken. The name of the EMT will appear elsewhere on the report. The arm used and position of the patient are not usually noted, but may be noted if the information is significant.

39. **c.** There should always be a minimum of two sets of vital signs recorded on every patient for the sake of comparison. A second set of vital signs should always be checked and compared for changes with the first set. The second set does not confirm the accuracy of the first set; it is an appropriate and important addition to a run report.

40. **a.** Vital signs on an unstable patient should be checked every 5 minutes. If the patient is stable, they should be checked every 15 minutes.

41. **d.** The letter "P" refers to "pertinent" past medical history, such as previous illnesses or injuries.

42. **a.** The letter "M" refers to the patient's present "medications."

43. **b.** The letter "E" relates to the "events" that led up to or caused the injury or illness.

44. **c.** The letter "L" refers to the patient's "last" oral intake, whether solids or liquids.

45. **d.** All of the above. The allergies an EMT is concerned with are allergies to medications, food, or environmental factors, such as pollen or insect stings.

46. **c.** A sign is something the EMT sees, feels, or hears. A symptom is something the patient tells the EMT. A syndrome is a collection of symptoms. The "S" in S-A-M-P-L-E refers to "signs and symptoms."

47.

symptom	chest pain
sign	cyanosis
sign	apnea
both	difficulty breathing
symptom	nausea
sign	sweating
sign	cool skin
symptom	headache
symptom	dizziness
sign	paleness
sign	deformed extremity
sign	vomiting
sign	swelling
symptom	double vision
symptom	numbness
sign	wheezing

CHAPTER
3

AIRWAY CONTROL
AND OXYGEN ADMINISTRATION

1. When filled, an "E" tank will hold approximately:
   a. 350 liters of oxygen
   b. 625 liters of oxygen
   c. 2000 liters of oxygen
   d. 3000 liters of oxygen

2. When an oxygen tank is filled, the normal pressure in the tank is approximately:
   a. 1000 psi
   b. 1400 psi
   c. 2000 psi
   d. 2800 psi

 3. A hydrostatic test should be conducted on a steel oxygen tank every:
   a. 2 years
   b. 5 years
   c. 8 years
   d. 12 years

 4. The date circled in Figure 3-1 is the date:
   a. the tank was manufactured
   b. for the next hydrostatic test
   c. the tank was placed in service
   d. of the last hydrostatic test

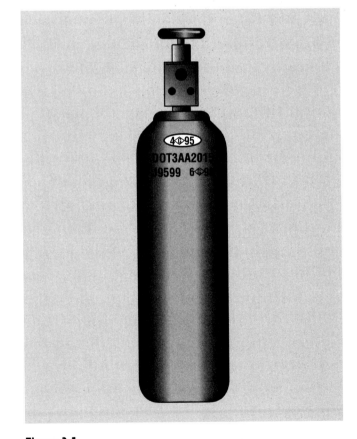

Figure 3-1

5. The safe working pressure of the tank in Figure 3-1 would be:
   a. 1500 psi
   b. 1750 psi
   c. 2015 psi
   d. 3000 psi

6. The tanks most commonly used in portable oxygen units are:
   a. "A" and "B" tanks
   b. "D" and "M" tanks
   c. "E" and "G" tanks
   d. "D" and "E" tanks

✳ 7. An oxygen regulator:
   a. increases pressure to 100 psi
   b. provides a constant flow rate of 25 lpm
   c. is needed only on oxygen tanks larger than "E" size
   d. reduces pressure to 40–70 psi

✳ 8. Pressure in an oxygen cylinder should not be allowed to drop below:
   a. 50 psi
   b. 200 psi
   c. 500 psi
   d. 1000 psi

9. To "crack" the valve of an oxygen tank means to:
   a. quickly open and close the valve to blow out dust
   b. strike the valve stem sharply with a metal object to loosen any dirt present in the valve opening
   c. damage the valve by dropping the tank
   d. seal the valve with tape after filling to prevent dust and dirt from entering it

10. When using supplemental oxygen with a pocket mask or bag-valve-mask, the proper flow rate is:
   a. less than 3 lpm if the patient has a history of respiratory illness
   b. 6 lpm
   c. 12 lpm
   d. 15 lpm

11. A nasal cannula will oxygenate patients:
   a. even if they breathe through their mouth
   b. only if they breathe through their nose
   c. as well as a complex mask
   d. even if a nasal obstruction is present

✳ 12. Oxygen may be administered to a laryngectomy patient by:
   a. inserting supply tubing into the stoma
   b. placing a cannula in the patient's nose
   c. placing a child or infant mask over the patient's stoma
   d. placing a mask on the patient and instructing the patient to breathe through the mouth only

13. Patients in shock due to trauma should be given oxygen:
   a. at a high-flow rate unless there is a history of asthma
   b. at a high-flow rate via a nonrebreather reservoir mask
   c. using the device best tolerated by the patient
   d. only after removal from a vehicle due to the potential of fire

14. The proper oxygen flow rate for a nonrebreather mask is:
   a. 3 lpm if there is a history of asthma
   b. 6 lpm if the patient will not tolerate high flow
   c. 9 lpm if the patient complains of a dry mouth
   d. 15 lpm in all cases

15. The reservoir of a nonrebreather mask should:
   a. fully deflate with each patient ventilation to allow the EMT to assess depth of breaths
   b. be inflated prior to placing the mask on the patient
   c. be filled with the patient's expired air
   d. be removed if the patient insists that he or she is not getting enough air

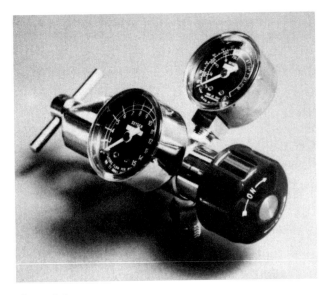

Figure 3-2

16. A nasal cannula can be used if:
  a. the patient will not tolerate a
     nonrebreather mask
  b. the patient complains of a dry mouth
  c. a low oxygen tank pressure is
     discovered
  d. the patient is breathing primarily
     through the nose

17. There is no advantage to using nasal
    cannulas with oxygen flow rates
    greater than:
  a. 2 lpm
  b. 4 lpm
  c. 6 lpm
  d. 9 lpm

*For questions 18–21, refer to Figures 3-2
and 3-3.*

 18. Figure 3-2 is an example of a:
  a. pressure-compensated flowmeter
  b. Bourdon gauge flowmeter
  c. ball valve flowmeter
  d. Thorpe tube-type flowmeter

 19. Figure 3-3 is an example of a:
  a. Bourdon gauge flowmeter
  b. ball valve flowmeter
  c. Venturi tube flowmeter
  d. pressure-compensated flowmeter

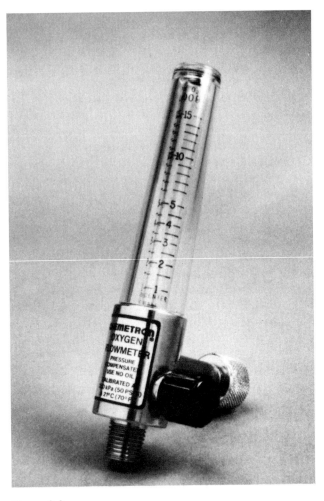

Figure 3-3

20. A disadvantage associated with the
    flowmeter in Figure 3-2 is that it:
  a. cannot be used with a "D" tank
  b. is difficult to operate
  c. does not compensate for back pressure
  d. cannot provide flow rates greater than
     5 lpm

21. A potential problem with the flowmeter in
    Figure 3-3 is that it:
  a. is affected by gravity
  b. cannot be used with on-board
     ambulance oxygen systems
  c. is not accurate
  d. cannot be used with infants or children

22. To administer oxygen to a conscious child who will not tolerate a mask, the EMT may need to:
   a. force it on the patient regardless of whether the child tolerates it
   b. administer oxygen using a blow-by technique to increase the concentration of the surrounding air
   c. place an adult mask over the child's entire face
   d. place a child mask tightly over the child's face and restrain the patient's hands

23. The airway that is least likely to stimulate vomiting in a semiconscious patient with an intact gag reflex is the:
   a. oropharyngeal airway
   b. nasopharyngeal airway
   c. esophageal obturator airway
   d. endotracheal airway

24. When a single rescuer is using a bag-valve-mask or a flow-restricted, oxygen-powered ventilation device, the EMT should:
   a. only use an adjunctive airway in adult patients
   b. only use an adjunctive airway for infants or children
   c. always use an adjunctive airway
   d. only use a nasopharyngeal airway

25. To determine the proper size of an oral airway to be inserted, measure from the:
   a. patient's Adam's apple to the corner of the mouth
   b. angle of the patient's jaw to the Adam's apple
   c. angle of the patient's jaw to the clavicle
   d. patient's earlobe to the corner of the mouth

26. To insert an oral airway in an adult, insert the airway:
   a. upside-down, then rotate it 180 degrees
   b. by pushing the tip along the tongue
   c. until the flange lies immediately behind the teeth
   d. so the flange lies 1 inch beyond the lips

27. When using a nasopharyngeal airway:
   a. lubricate the airway with petroleum jelly before inserting
   b. size the airway by measuring from the tip of the nose to the tip of the patient's ear
   c. force the tube if resistance is met
   d. do not try the other nostril if resistance is met when attempting insertion

28. If a patient is not breathing, the EMT should:
   a. immediately begin ventilating with an appropriate ventilation device
   b. wait until oxygen is available to begin ventilation
   c. delay ventilation until an adjunctive airway is available
   d. never ventilate an adult patient at a rate greater than 12 times per minute

29. The EMT should assist with ventilation of an adult patient if the breathing rate falls below:
   a. 8 breaths per minute
   b. 12 breaths per minute
   c. 14 breaths per minute
   d. 16 breaths per minute

30. A bag-valve-mask should be connected to oxygen:
   a. only if the patient is cyanotic
   b. only when ventilating infants or children
   c. only if the patient has no history of breathing problems
   d. whenever it is available

31. The advantage of using a flow-restricted, oxygen-powered ventilation device versus a bag-valve-mask is that:
   a. an oral or nasal airway is not needed
   b. it does not need a mask
   c. it is easier to use with one rescuer
   d. it requires no training to use

32. A flow-restricted, oxygen-powered ventilation device should *not* be used on:
   a. infants or small children
   b. any trauma patient
   c. patients who are breathing
   d. patients without a gag reflex

33. A flow-restricted, oxygen-powered ventilation device:
a. can be used if the oxygen tank becomes empty
b. provides only 60% oxygen
c. provides flow rates of 20 lpm
d. may produce gastric distention due to the high pressure of the oxygen delivered

✱ 34. A major problem associated with the use of a bag-valve-mask is:
a. difficulty maintaining a good seal with the mask
b. inability to deliver an adequate concentration of oxygen
c. inability to see if the patient has vomited
d. that it is difficult for two operators to use

✱ 35. If a patient with an oral airway in place becomes conscious and develops a gag reflex:
a. restrain the patient and keep the airway in place
b. remove the airway and suction the patient if necessary
c. remove the airway and insert a smaller one
d. replace the oral airway with an endotracheal tube

36. A suction unit should provide a vacuum of:
a. no more than 100 mm Hg of negative pressure
b. no more than 200 mm Hg of negative pressure
c. no less than 300 mm Hg of negative pressure
d. no less than 400 mm Hg of negative pressure

37. Two common types of suction catheters used by EMTs are:
a. hard and rigid
b. French and soft
c. hard and soft
d. English and tonsil tip

38. When suctioning a patient, the EMT should:
a. insert the catheter without suction
b. suction only while advancing the catheter
c. not be concerned with wearing gloves, as there should be no physical contact with the patient
d. be careful not to rotate the catheter

39. The maximum length of time that an EMT should suction a patient is:
a. 5 seconds at a time
b. 15 seconds at a time
c. 20 seconds at a time
d. 25 seconds at a time

40. A suction catheter should not be inserted farther than the:
a. larynx
b. first set of molars
c. trachea
d. base of the tongue

ADDITIONAL POINTS FOR DISCUSSION

1. At what point does your service refill or replace its portable or on-board oxygen tanks?

2. What is your department's procedure for refilling or replacing oxygen tanks?

3. How would you handle a situation in which multiple patients require mass oxygen administration?

4. Review the operation of your department's on-board and portable suction units.

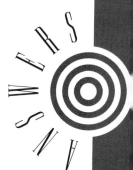
3 AIRWAY CONTROL AND OXYGEN ADMINISTRATION

1. b. An "E" tank will hold approximately 625 liters of oxygen when filled. A "D" tank will hold 350 liters, and an "M" tank will hold 3000 liters.

2. c. The pressure in a full oxygen tank is approximately 2000 psi.

3. b. Steel oxygen tanks should be hydrostatically tested every 5 years. Although some sources say aluminum oxygen tanks need to be tested only every 10 years, it is recommended that aluminum tanks also be tested every 5 years.

4. d. The date circled is the date of the last hydrostatic test.

5. c. The tank's safe working pressure is 2015 psi. This corresponds to the last four digits of the first line stamped on the tank in Figure 3-1.

6. d. "D" and "E" tanks are most commonly used in portable oxygen units. "M" and "G" tanks are commonly used for on-board ambulance oxygen systems.

7. d. The first stage of an oxygen regulator reduces the pressure of the oxygen coming from the cylinder to 40–70 psi.

8. b. The pressure of an oxygen tank should not fall below 200 psi. This is also called the safe residual pressure. Allowing the pressure to drop below this point may allow moisture and dirt to enter the tank, which may cause rust in steel tanks. Many departments refill portable oxygen tanks long before reaching the safe residual pressure to ensure an adequate supply of oxygen at an emergency scene.

9. a. To "crack" the valve of an oxygen tank, quickly open and close the valve before attaching the regulator to the tank. This blows any dust or dirt out of the valve, thereby protecting the regulator from foreign matter that could compromise its operation.

10. d. When using supplemental oxygen with a pocket mask or bag-valve-mask, the flowmeter should be set at 15 lpm. If a pocket mask without an oxygen inlet is all that is available, a nasal cannula may be worn by the rescuer performing ventilation to increase the concentration of delivered oxygen.

11. a. A nasal cannula will oxygenate a patient even if they breathe through their mouth, provided they have a patent nasopharynx. This is because the oropharynx acts as a reservoir for the oxygen being delivered, thereby enriching the concentration of oxygen of the air breathed through the mouth. Patients with nasal obstructions, however, receive little benefit from use of a nasal cannula.

12. c. A child or infant mask may be placed over the stoma of a laryngectomy patient to provide supplemental oxygen. The use of a humidifier is recommended because the oxygen bypasses the normal structures of the nose and throat, which would naturally humidify the oxygen.

13. b. Any patient in shock, especially shock due to trauma, should receive a high-flow rate of oxygen via a nonrebreather mask. This is true even if the patient has a history of breathing problems such as emphysema. Early administration is important. Do not wait for victim removal to start giving oxygen.

14. d. The proper flow rate of oxygen for a nonrebreather mask is 15 lpm in all cases.

15. b. The reservoir of a nonrebreather mask allows delivery of high concentrations of oxygen. The reservoir should be filled with oxygen prior to placing the mask on the patient. If the reservoir deflates completely with each patient breath, the oxygen flow rate to the mask is too low and should be increased. There are no circumstances under which the reservoir should be removed.

16. a. The nasal cannula should only be used when a patient will not tolerate a nonrebreather mask despite reassurances from EMTs that adequate oxygen is being delivered.

17. c. When using a nasal cannula, flow rates greater than 6 lpm are of little value.

18. b. A Bourdon gauge flowmeter is shown in Figure 3-2.

19. d. A pressure-compensated flowmeter is shown in Figure 3-3.

20. c. The flowmeter in Figure 3-2 does not compensate for back pressure. It is, however, commonly used on portable oxygen systems as it provides high flow rates and is easy to use.

21. a. The disadvantage of the flowmeter in Figure 3-3 is that it is affected by gravity. It must be used in an upright position, and is very accurate when used correctly. Although this type of flowmeter is not good for use with portable oxygen systems, it does work well with on-board systems.

22. b. To administer oxygen to a conscious child who will not tolerate a mask, use a blow-by technique. This may be accomplished through various methods. Oxygen tubing can be held about 2 inches from the patient's face, or it may be inserted into a paper cup held near the child's face. Or, an oxygen mask may be held near the child's face. The objective is to increase the concentration of oxygen in the surrounding air. A good indication of how badly the child needs oxygen is whether he or she will accept it. Seriously ill or injured infants and children usually do not fight the oxygen mask.

23. b. A nasopharyngeal airway, although often overlooked by EMTs, is better tolerated in a semiconscious patient with a gag reflex. Oral airways and endotracheal tubes can only be used when the gag reflex is absent or deeply depressed.

24. **c.** An adjunctive airway should always be used when ventilating a patient with a flow-restricted, oxygen-powered ventilation device or when a single rescuer is using a bag-valve-mask. Various airways are available for use with patients of all ages.

25. **d.** Measuring from the patient's earlobe to the corner of the mouth will provide a useful guide for sizing an oral airway. The EMT can also measure from the corner of the patient's mouth to the angle of the jaw.

26. **a.** To place an oral airway in an adult, insert it upside-down and then rotate it 180 degrees. An alternate method is to use a tongue depressor to manage the tongue while inserting the airway right-side up.

27. **b.** A nasopharyngeal airway may be sized by measuring from the tip of the patient's nose to the tip of the ear. Do not use petroleum jelly or other non–water-based lubricants on the airway. If resistance is met, do not force the airway; instead, try the other nostril.

28. **a.** If a patient is not breathing, the EMT should immediately begin ventilating with an appropriate ventilation device. Although an airway and oxygen should be used as soon as possible with such patients, the EMT should not delay ventilation to wait for either. The ventilation rate does not have to be limited to 12 times a minute. Patients in need of oxygen should be hyperventilated in the early stages of ventilatory management.

29. **a.** As a general rule, if a patient's breathing rate falls below eight breaths a minute, the EMT should assist breathing. Some patients with higher breathing rates may also need assistance. Decisions should be based on the patient's overall condition, not simply the breathing rate.

30. **d.** Although a bag-valve-mask can be used with room air, supplemental oxygen should be connected to the device whenever it is available. Also, an oxygen reservoir should always be attached. In essence, the bag-valve-mask should be considered a multipart system, and all components (i.e., the bag-valve-mask, oxygen reservoir, and tubing) should be stored together.

31. **c.** The advantage of using a flow-restricted, oxygen-powered ventilation device over a bag-valve-mask is that it is easier for a single rescuer to use. The device uses the same type of mask as a bag-valve-mask, and an airway should be used. EMTs need training to properly use the device.

32. **a.** Flow-restricted, oxygen-powered ventilation devices should not be used on infants or small children (consult local protocols for exact age criteria). They can be used on some trauma patients and in patients without a gag reflex. The device may be used to support ventilation in a patient who is breathing.

33. **d.** The pressure generated with a flow-restricted, oxygen-powered ventilation device may cause gastric distention; they deliver 100% oxygen at flow rates of 40 lpm. Such devices will not operate if the oxygen tank becomes empty.

34. **a.** The major problem associated with a bag-valve-mask, especially when it is used by one rescuer, is the inability to maintain a good seal with the mask to ensure adequate ventilation. This problem can be lessened if two EMTs use the device, with one maintaining a mask seal and the other squeezing the bag. Bag-valve-masks are capable of delivering high concentrations of oxygen. Clear face masks should be used so the EMT can see if the patient vomits.

35. b. If a patient with an oral airway in place develops a gag reflex, remove the airway and suction the patient if necessary.

36. c. Suction units should provide no less than 300 mm Hg of negative pressure.

37. c. The hard suction catheter (also known as a rigid catheter, tonsil tip, tonsil sucker, or Yankauer) and soft suction catheter (also known as a French catheter) are both commonly used by EMTs.

38. a. When suctioning a patient, insert the catheter without suction. Suction should be applied only while withdrawing the catheter. Rotating the catheter between the fingers with a twirling motion will keep the tip from sticking to the tissue and will cover all areas being suctioned. The EMT should wear gloves while suctioning.

39. b. A patient should not be suctioned for longer than 15 seconds at a time. The goal of suctioning a patient's airway is to clear the airway. Remember, however, that while suctioning fluids, the EMT is also suctioning oxygen. It may be necessary to suction the patient a number of times to thoroughly clear the airway. Oxygenate the patient between each suctioning period.

40. d. A suction catheter should not be inserted farther than the base of the patient's tongue.

PATIENT ASSESSMENT

1. Evaluation of the scene:
   a. includes taking appropriate body substance isolation measures
   b. is only necessary when a trauma scene is being approached
   c. should be done immediately following initial patient assessment
   d. should be performed by the senior EMT on the crew

2. If a scene is not safe and the EMT cannot make it safe:
   a. enter only if the patient's life is in immediate danger
   b. do not enter
   c. one EMT should enter while another stands by for assistance to arrive
   d. return to the station until the scene becomes safe

3. When an injured patient is found at a crime scene:
   a. have the police bring the patient to the EMTs in order for them to provide patient care
   b. wait to begin patient care until law enforcement officials have completed their investigation
   c. be careful about disturbing the scene while providing patient care
   d. immediately move the patient to the ambulance prior to providing any care

4. Match the following injuries with the mechanism that is most likely to have caused the injury:
   chest injury, head/cervical spine injury, hip injury
   _____ windshield broken in a spiderweb pattern
   _____ broken car dashboard
   _____ accident in the shallow end of a swimming pool
   _____ bent steering wheel or steering column

5. The initial assessment includes the EMT's general impression of the patient and evaluating, in order, the patient's:
   a. mental status, airway, breathing, and circulation
   b. level of consciousness, blood pressure, and pulse
   c. airway, pulse, blood pressure, and responsiveness
   d. pulse, bleeding, airway, and family history

6. When a life-threatening condition is discovered during the initial assessment:
   a. immediately skip to a focused trauma history
   b. note the condition and correct it during the appropriate part of the detailed exam
   c. deal with the condition immediately
   d. note the condition on the run report and let the hospital deal with it

7. Cervical spine stabilization should first be accomplished:
   a. while the secondary survey is being performed
   b. after the patient is log-rolled onto the backboard
   c. when the patient's mental status is being assessed
   d. after the vital signs have been checked

8. When using the AVPU scale for noting a patient's level of consciousness, "V" would signify that the patient:
   a. is "vocal" and able to speak
   b. responds to "verbal" stimuli
   c. responds to "visual" stimuli
   d. has spontaneous "ventilations"

9. The letter "P" in AVPU refers to whether the patient:
   a. is oriented to "place"
   b. is a "priority" patient
   c. has a "pulse"
   d. responds to "painful" stimuli

10. When assessing mental status, it is important to note:
   a. precisely how the patient answers the questions
   b. whether the patient is intoxicated
   c. any changes for the better or worse
   d. all of the above

11. The problem with asking a vehicle crash patient, "Where are you?" to check the level of consciousness is:
   a. the patient really may not know where he or she is
   b. street signs may be missing
   c. the EMTs may not know where they are
   d. it does not stimulate enough thinking

12. When checking a patient's orientation to place, person, purpose, and time, the last thing the patient will normally forget is:
   a. place
   b. person
   c. purpose
   d. time

13. A legitimate reason for an EMT to search the wallet of an unconscious patient is:
   a. to look for pertinent medical information, such as a medical alert card
   b. to look for illegal drugs that may be involved
   c. to remove money for safekeeping
   d. all of the above

14. To open the airway of an unresponsive trauma patient, use the:
   a. chin lift
   b. head tilt
   c. modified jaw thrust
   d. neck lift

15. Maintaining adequate breathing in a trauma patient includes:
   a. placing the patient in a pneumatic antishock garment (PASG)
   b. placing the patient in the shock position
   c. sealing open chest wounds
   d. sitting the patient upright

16. When examining a severely injured or unconscious multisystem trauma patient, it is important to:
   a. remove as little of the patient's clothing as possible
   b. remove all the patient's clothing
   c. remove clothing only around areas of obvious injury or pain
   d. remove no clothing, as this may cause hypothermia

17. An important part of assessing circulation in all patients includes:
   a. checking the femoral pulse
   b. placing the patient on a backboard
   c. checking for capillary refill time
   d. evaluating for major bleeding

18. Fill in each blank of the following list with a **Y** (for yes) or **N** (for no) regarding whether the patient would be considered a priority patient:

___ Unresponsive patient without a gag reflex

___ Pregnant female patient in labor with no complications

___ Elderly male patient complaining of feeling tired

___ 48-year-old male patient with chest pain and a blood pressure of 90/60

___ 19-year-old female patient with a severe leg laceration that is bleeding uncontrollably

___ 16-year-old female patient who experienced chest pain an hour ago but has no pain now

___ Patient having severe difficulty breathing

___ Patient experiencing signs of hypoperfusion

___ Pregnant female patient with breech birth presentation

___ Patient with a painful, swollen, deformed extremity with good distal pulses

___ Patient experiencing severe abdominal pain

___ Conscious patient who is disoriented and does not follow commands

___ Patient complaining of nausea and vomiting

___ Diabetic patient who was weak and light-headed but claims to feel fine after drinking sweetened orange juice

___ Driver of a vehicle struck from the rear by another vehicle at low speed complaining of upper back and neck pain

19. When a priority patient is identified:
    a. call for Advanced Life Support assistance and wait at the scene
    b. expedite transport to an appropriate medical facility
    c. call medical control and request further instructions for on-scene management
    d. immediately transport the patient to the hospital that he or she has requested

20. When an EMT encounters a patient from a vehicle where an air bag was deployed:
    a. there is little chance of the patient having received significant injury
    b. the patient is fine if he or she appears stable after the first 5–10 minutes
    c. check the patient for steam burns
    d. lift the air bag and check the steering wheel for deformity

21. A rapid trauma assessment should be performed on:
    a. any unresponsive trauma patient
    b. all trauma patients
    c. any patient complaining of neck pain
    d. any patient with a painful, swollen, deformed extremity

22. A rapid trauma assessment is a:
    a. rapid evaluation of the patient's airway and cervical spine
    b. methodical exam limited to the area of injury
    c. rapid examination of the mechanism of injury and scene
    d. quick head-to-toe exam

23. A rapid trauma assessment should be performed in:
    a. 10–30 seconds
    b. 30–60 seconds
    c. 60–90 seconds
    d. 90–120 seconds

24. When a multisystem trauma patient is encountered:
    a. deal with life-threatening conditions first
    b. focus on the patient's most painful injury first
    c. focus on the injury that appears the worst first
    d. do not manage any injuries until the rapid trauma assessment is complete

Questions 25–32 involve the acronym DCAP-BTLS as it relates to assessment.

25. The letter "L" refers to the presence of:
a. "light-headedness"
b. "lacerations"
c. "lethargy"
d. "liquids" coming from the ears or nose

26. During the "C" portion, check the patient for:
a. "cardiac" problems
b. "chest" injuries
c. "contusions"
d. "carotid" pulses

27. "S" represents:
a. "sweating"
b. "skin" color
c. "swelling"
d. "severity" of injuries

28. "B" relates to:
a. checking the patient's "back"
b. "backboarding" the patient
c. assessing the patient's "breathing"
d. checking for "burns"

29. The letter "D" refers to:
a. "dizziness"
b. "deformities"
c. "difficulty" breathing
d. "distal" pulses

30. "T" reminds the EMT to:
a. assess the patient's "trachea"
b. check for loose "teeth"
c. look for "tenderness"
d. question the patient about "time"

31. The letter "P" is connected with:
a. "penetrations or punctures"
b. "pain"
c. checking the patient's "pulse"
d. whether a female patient is "pregnant"

32. "A" refers to the presence of:
a. "airway" problems
b. "avulsions"
c. "allergies"
d. "abrasions"

33. When assessing the patient's neck, the EMT should look for:
a. carotid artery retention
b. laryngospasms
c. jugular vein distention
d. tracheal transfixation

34. The term used to describe the unusual, opposite motion of a section of chest wall that may be noted on a patient with a serious chest injury is:
a. paroxysmal movement
b. oppositional motion
c. paradoxical motion
d. inordinate movement

35. If a conscious trauma patient is complaining of severe pain in the pelvic region:
a. do not flex or compress the pelvic girdle
b. compress the pelvic region to see if compression elicits further pain
c. log-roll the patient onto his or her side and assess the posterior pelvis
d. have the patient move his or her legs into a position that relieves the pain

36. Evaluation of the adult patient's extremities involves checking for DCAP-BTLS and:
a. capillary refill, sensation, and circulation
b. circulation, motor function, and sensation
c. reflexes, pulses, and color
d. blood pressure, reflexes, and motor function

37. An often-overlooked but important part of the focused history and physical exam section of the trauma assessment involves checking the patient's:
    a. posterior body
    b. airway
    c. reflexes
    d. mental status

38. If only one EMT is present, the rapid trauma assessment should be performed:
    a. before the initial assessment
    b. after baseline vital signs and history are obtained
    c. before any cervical spine precautions are taken
    d. after an initial assessment is done

39. When managing a patient with single-system trauma, such as a lacerated arm, the focused history and physical examination should begin:
    a. at the head, working toward the injury
    b. at the site of the injury
    c. with reevaluation of the airway
    d. with cervical immobilization

40. When the EMT encounters an unresponsive medical patient, the next step after the initial assessment is:
    a. an assessment of the chest to evaluate the lungs and heart
    b. a detailed physical exam
    c. a rapid head-to-toe assessment similar to the rapid trauma assessment
    d. an abbreviated focused history

41. The assessment of a responsive medical patient:
    a. emphasizes the patient's vital signs
    b. is not as critical as that of an unresponsive patient if there is no previous history of medical problems
    c. can usually wait until the patient is moved to the ambulance
    d. is normally based on the patient's primary complaint

Questions 42–47 refer to the acronym O-P-Q-R-S-T.

42. The letter "O" refers to:
    a. the patient's last "oral" intake
    b. whether the patient is "oriented"
    c. the time of "onset" of the problem
    d. performing an "ongoing" assessment

43. The letter "P" relates to:
    a. severity of "pain"
    b. "provocation"
    c. what the main "problem" is
    d. the "primary" complaint

44. The letter "Q" refers to:
    a. how "quickly" the problem started
    b. the "quality" of the pain
    c. the "quantity" of medications regularly taken by the patient
    d. whether the patient "qualifies" as a priority patient

45. The letter "R" component involves asking the patient if:
    a. anything provides "relief" of the pain
    b. this is a "regular" problem
    c. the onset of the problem was "rapid"
    d. the pain "radiates" to other areas

46. The letter "S" is associated with:
    a. "symptoms"
    b. "severity"
    c. "signs"
    d. "sensation"

47. The letter "T" refers to:
    a. "time"
    b. the patient's "temperature"
    c. whether the problem involves "trauma"
    d. the "type" of problem

48. When an unresponsive patient is encountered:
a. O-P-Q-R-S-T information cannot be obtained
b. it is not important to gain O-P-Q-R-S-T information
c. O-P-Q-R-S-T information may be obtained from family, friends, or bystanders
d. accurate O-P-Q-R-S-T information can only be obtained if the patient regains consciousness

49. The detailed physical exam is a:
a. rapid neurologic exam
b. breathing and pulse check
c. 15-minute thorough exam limited to the injured body system
d. a methodical head-to-toe examination

50. The primary purpose of the detailed physical exam is to:
a. check for signs of physical abuse or drug use
b. find less serious hidden injuries or medical problems
c. confirm that a medical problem exists
d. help the EMT diagnose the patient's problem

51. Of the following, the patient who would not need a complete and thorough detailed physical exam is:
a. an unresponsive medical patient
b. a trauma patient with an altered mental status
c. a patient with a history of heart problems who is complaining of mild chest pain
d. a patient who was ejected from a vehicle but is complaining only of shoulder pain

✱ 52. A major part of the detailed physical exam assesses:
a. O-P-Q-R-S-T
b. S-A-M-P-L-E history
c. DCAP-BTLS
d. A-B-Cs

53. When checking the patient's ears, the EMT should be alert for the presence of blood mixed with:
a. vitreous fluid
b. cerebrospinal fluid
c. synovial fluid
d. lacrimal fluid

54. When assessing the patient's chest:
a. look for paradoxical movement
b. check breath sounds
c. feel for crepitation
d. all of the above

✱ 55. Wheezing can be described as a:
a. harsh, raspy sound created by fluid in the lungs
b. crowing sound heard on inspiration
c. fine, crackling sound indicating the presence of fluid in the small airways
d. high-pitched, whistling sound created as air flows through narrowed airways

✱ 56. When assessing the abdomen:
a. inform the patient prior to palpating
b. do not let the patient know you are going to palpate
c. feel only in the area of discomfort
d. press as deeply as possible

57. Ideally, the detailed physical exam should be performed:
a. while the patient is still in the house
b. prior to leaving for the hospital
c. after Advanced Life Support personnel arrive
d. en route to the hospital

58. During the ongoing assessment:
a. assure adequacy of oxygen delivery and artificial ventilation, and the adequacy of EMT interventions
b. repeat a head-to-toe exam
c. record the vital signs and S-A-M-P-L-E history every 10 minutes
d. perform a detailed physical exam

59. A stable patient should receive an ongoing assessment every:
a. 5 minutes
b. 10 minutes
c. 15 minutes
d. 20 minutes

60. In essence, the ongoing assessment repeats all the components of the:
a. detailed physical exam
b. initial assessment
c. rapid trauma assessment
d. S-A-M-P-L-E history

61. An important component of patient assessment that must not be neglected is:
a. providing emotional reassurance to the patient
b. obtaining insurance information for billing purposes
c. passing information on to law enforcement officers
d. telling the patient everything will be all right

If your training includes the use of the Glasgow Coma Scale when assessing patients, complete questions 62–64. Refer to the Glasgow Coma Scale in Figure 4-1.

62. Your patient is a 30-year-old man who is lying on the sidewalk. His eyes are closed, and he opens them only on voice command. He can speak, but his answers are inaccurate. During the exam, he reacts to pain by attempting to push your hand away from the painful area. His Glasgow Coma Scale score is:
a. 11
b. 12
c. 13
d. 14

1. **Eye opening**	Points	
● Spontaneous	4	
● To voice	3	
● To pain	2	
● None	1	____
2. **Verbal response**	Points	
● Oriented	5	
● Confused	4	
● Inappropriate words	3	
● Incomprehensible words	2	
● None	1	____
3. **Motor responses**	Points	
● Obeys commands	6	
● Purposeful movement (pain)	5	
● Withdrawal (pain)	4	
● Flexion (pain)	3	
● Extension (pain)	2	
● None	1	____
Total (1 + 2 + 3)		____

Figure 4-1 Glasgow Coma Scale.

63. A semiconscious hit-and-run patient is found lying next to the road. She does not open her eyes in response to any stimulus. She does respond to painful stimuli by groaning and moving her arms away from the source of pain. Her Glasgow Coma Scale score is:
a. 5
b. 6
c. 7
d. 8

64. A Glasgow Coma Scale score that would be considered normal is:
a. 9–10
b. 11–12
c. 14–15
d. 17–18

ADDITIONAL POINTS FOR DISCUSSION

1. Many Emergency Medical Services have a number of hospitals to which they may transport their patients. Some of these medical facilities are specially equipped and staffed to handle certain types of emergencies. It is important for EMTs to be aware of the special skills or limitations of each hospital they use.

To what hospitals or medical facilities in your area would you normally transport the following type of patient:

* Multisystem trauma?

* Critical burns?

* Major head injury or neurologic problems?

* Unstable cardiac problems?

* Critical obstetric emergencies?

* Contamination from a radiation or hazardous materials incident?

* Amputation or severe avulsion that may be surgically reattached?

2. If your service is a Basic Life Support service, is Advanced Life Support available from another service? When would you call for Advanced Life Support assistance?

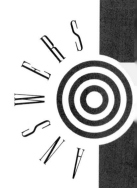

4 PATIENT ASSESSMENT

1. **a.** Scene evaluation includes taking appropriate body substance isolation measures. This should be done on all calls. The EMT must determine whether the scene is safe prior to assessing the patient. Everyone on the crew is responsible for looking for unsafe situations.

2. **b.** If a scene is not safe and the EMT cannot make it safe, do not enter the scene. Remember, dead EMTs don't save lives.

3. **c.** An injured patient at a crime scene still needs medical attention. However, try to disturb the scene as little as possible. The EMT must be careful not to be in such a hurry to move the patient that further harm is done to the patient.

4.
head/cervical spine injury	windshield broken in a spiderweb pattern
hip injury	broken car dashboard
head/cervical spine injury	accident in the shallow end of a swimming pool
chest injury	bent steering wheel or steering column

5. **a.** The initial assessment includes the EMT's general impressions of the patient and assessing the patient's mental status, airway, breathing, and circulation.

6. **c.** When a life-threatening condition is discovered during the initial assessment, it should be dealt with immediately.

7. **c.** Cervical spine stabilization should take place while the patient's mental status is being assessed.

8. **b.** The letter "V" signifies the patient responds to "verbal" stimuli, "A" corresponds to "alert," and "U" means the patient is "unresponsive" to any stimuli.

9. **d.** The letter "P" refers to whether the patient responds to "painful" stimuli.

10. **c.** When assessing mental status, it is important to note any changes for the better or worse. Changes are important as they act as a baseline for comparison. The patient's answers don't need to be written verbatim. Although a patient may appear to be intoxicated, even someone who has been drinking may have underlying trauma or a medical problem affecting their mental status.

11. **a.** The problem with asking a vehicle crash patient "Where are you?" or "Do you know where you are?" is that many times the patient may be alert and yet not know where he or she is. A better question to ask, especially to the elderly, is "Do you know where you were going?"

12. b. Normally, the last thing a patient forgets is "person," that is, who they are. That is because this information is stored in long-term memory. Short-term memory, such as where they are (place), time, and what they were doing (purpose) immediately prior to the event, will be forgotten first.

13. a. Looking for pertinent medical information is the only legitimate reason for an EMT to search a patient's wallet.

14. c. Use the modified jaw thrust to open the airway of an unresponsive trauma patient.

15. c. Open chest wounds compromise the lung's ability to function; therefore, they must be sealed with an occlusive dressing to maintain adequate breathing. Sitting a trauma patient upright is contraindicated due to the possibility of cervical spine injury. Placing the patient in a PASG or the shock position will not assure a patent airway.

16. b. It is generally recommended that the EMT remove all clothing from a seriously injured multisystem trauma patient, especially if the patient is unconscious and cannot verbally communicate. In many cases, it is not the injuries you see that will kill the patient, but the ones you don't see. Discretion should be exercised to keep embarrassment to a minimum. Because it can be avoided by using blankets, hypothermia is not a valid reason to leave clothing in place.

17. d. While assessing circulation, the EMT should check for and correct major bleeding.

18. Fill in each blank of the following list with a **Y** (for yes) or **N** (for no) regarding whether the patient would be considered a priority patient:

   Y   Unresponsive patient without a gag reflex

   N   Pregnant female patient in labor with no complications

   N   Elderly male patient complaining of feeling tired

   Y   48-year-old male patient with chest pain and a blood pressure of 90/60

   Y   19-year-old female patient with a severe leg laceration that is bleeding uncontrollably

   N   16-year-old female patient who experienced chest pain an hour ago but has no pain now

   Y   Patient with severe difficulty breathing

   Y   Patient experiencing signs of hypoperfusion

   Y   Pregnant female patient with breech birth presentation

   N   Patient with a painful, swollen, deformed extremity with good distal pulses

   Y   Patient experiencing severe abdominal pain

   Y   Conscious patient who is disoriented and does not follow commands

   N   Patient complaining of nausea and vomiting

   N   Diabetic patient who was weak and light-headed but claims to feel fine after drinking sweetened orange juice

   N   Driver of a vehicle struck from the rear by another vehicle at low speed complaining of upper back and neck pain

19. b. When a priority patient is identified, expedite transport to an appropriate medical facility. If Advanced Life Support is available, it should be requested. However, do not delay transport for the arrival of an Advanced Life Support unit.

20. **d.** Although air bags can reduce the incidence of injuries from vehicle crashes, they can still cause harm to a patient. A patient may sustain an injury yet not show immediate signs of the injury. If an air bag has been deployed, lift the air bag and check the steering wheel for deformity or damage. If either is noted, suspect injury to the patient.

21. **a.** A rapid trauma assessment should be performed on any unresponsive trauma patient as well as any trauma patient who has a significant mechanism of injury.

22. **d.** A rapid trauma assessment is a quick head-to-toe exam.

23. **c.** A rapid trauma assessment should be performed in 60–90 seconds.

24. **a.** When a multisystem trauma patient is encountered, deal with life-threatening conditions first. Do not be fooled into focusing on the patient's most painful injury or the worst-appearing injury first.

25. **b.** "L" refers to "lacerations."

26. **c.** "C" involves checking for "contusions."

27. **c.** "S" represents "swelling."

28. **d.** "B" relates to checking for "burns."

29. **b.** "D" refers to "deformities."

30. **c.** "T" should remind the EMT to look for "tenderness."

31. **a.** "P" is connected with penetrations or "punctures."

32. **d.** "A" refers to abrasions.

33. **c.** When examining the neck, look for jugular vein distention. The veins in the neck will be abnormally enlarged.

34. **c.** Paradoxical motion refers to the unusual, opposite motion of a section of chest wall that may be seen when a patient sustains serious chest injury. The section of chest wall moves inward as the rest of the chest moves outward on inspiration, and outward as the rest of the chest moves inward on exhalation.

35. **a.** If a conscious trauma patient is complaining of severe pain in the pelvic region, do not flex or compress the pelvic girdle, as this may cause further injury. If the patient is unconscious, checking the stability of the pelvis is warranted. Do not log-roll or move the legs of a patient with a suspected pelvic injury.

36. **b.** Evaluation of the patient's extremities includes checking circulation (distal pulses), motor function, and sensation.

37. **a.** Many EMTs often forget to check a patient's posterior body during the trauma assessment. Life-threatening injuries may be missed if this important part of the patient exam is neglected. The airway is checked during the initial assessment. Reflexes are not checked by EMTs.

38. **d.** If only one EMT is present, the rapid trauma assessment should be performed after an initial assessment is done. Vital signs and history are taken after the rapid assessment. Although it may be difficult when only one EMT is present, cervical spine precautions should still be taken to the best extent possible before the rapid trauma assessment is performed. If two EMTs are present, some procedures can be performed at the same time.

39. b. When managing a patient with single system trauma, such as a lacerated arm, the focused history and physical examination should begin at the site of the injury. However, if the patient appears confused or if there is a significant mechanism of injury, a complete head-to-toe exam is necessary.

40. c. When the EMT encounters an unresponsive medical patient, a rapid head-to-toe assessment similar to the rapid trauma assessment should be done after the initial assessment.

41. d. The assessment of a responsive medical patient is normally based on the patient's primary complaint. Do not delay assessment until the patient is in the ambulance. If assessment is delayed, management of the patient, such as assisting with medications, may also be delayed.

42. c. The letter "O" refers to the time of "onset" of the problem. This is when the medical problem first started, and may be a short or long period prior to when the EMS was called.

43. b. The letter "P" stands for "provocation," that is, what made the pain start or what makes it worse.

44. b. The letter "Q" refers to the "quality" of the pain. This is a description of the characteristics of the discomfort, such as whether the pain is sharp, dull, or stabbing, or whether it is a constant or intermittent pressure.

45. d. The letter "R" involves asking the patient if the pain "radiates" to other areas of the body.

46. b. The letter "S" is associated with "severity."

47. a. The letter "T" refers to "time." Time primarily relates to duration of the pain, such as if the pain has been going on for some time, or if it has gotten better, then worse. It is also important to note if there was a particular time when the problem got worse and prompted the patient to finally call EMS.

48. c. When the EMT encounters an unresponsive patient, O-P-Q-R-S-T information may be obtained from family, friends, or bystanders.

49. d. The detailed physical exam is a methodical head-to-toe examination. Although it covers many items that were checked in the rapid trauma assessment, the detailed exam is slower, methodical, and more comprehensive. It expands upon the assessment steps in the focused history and physical examination.

50. b. The primary purpose of the detailed physical exam is to find less serious hidden injuries or medical problems.

51. c. A patient with a history of heart problems who is complaining of mild chest pain would not need a detailed physical exam because little information is likely to be gained from palpating every body part of this patient. This would also be true of a patient with minor single-system trauma, such as a foot laceration. A detailed physical exam should be performed on any unresponsive medical or trauma patient, patients with altered mental status, or patients with a significant mechanism of injury involved.

52. c. A major part of the detailed physical exam assesses DCAP-BTLS.

53. b. Check for cerebrospinal fluid when checking the ears. If blood is also present, place some on a 4 × 4 gauze pad. If cerebrospinal fluid is mixed with the blood, it will form a halo-like ring of fluid around the blood in the middle.

54. d. All of the above. Check breath sounds when assessing the patient's chest. Note whether they are present or absent, and equal or unequal. Also, look for paradoxical movement and feel for crepitation.

55. d. Wheezing can be described as a high-pitched, whistling sound created as air flows through narrowed airways.

56. a. When the abdomen is being assessed, inform the patient prior to palpating. Otherwise, the patient may be surprised and tighten the abdominal muscles. Do not begin in the immediate area of pain, if there is any. The EMT does not need to press deeply to note whether the abdomen is soft, firm, or distended.

57. d. Ideally, the detailed physical exam should be performed in the back of the ambulance en route to the hospital.

58. a. During the ongoing assessment, assure adequacy of oxygen delivery and artificial ventilation, as well as the adequacy of EMT interventions, such as checking dressings and splints.

59. c. A stable patient should receive an ongoing assessment every 15 minutes. An unstable patient should be reassessed every 5 minutes or less.

60. b. In essence, the ongoing assessment repeats all the components of the initial assessment.

61. a. An important component of patient assessment that must not be neglected is providing emotional reassurance to the patient. Often, patients are distraught and worried about their condition. The EMT can help to alleviate some of the anxiety. However, do not tell the patient everything will be all right, as this may not be the case.

62. b. The patient's score is 12: eye opening = 3, verbal response = 4, motor response = 5.

63. c. The patient's score is 7: eye opening = 1, verbal response = 2, motor response = 4.

64. c. A normal total score is 14–15. A patient's condition is considered serious when the score is less than 13.

CHAPTER 5

MEDICAL EMERGENCIES I

GENERAL PHARMACOLOGY

1. Four routes by which an EMT administers or assists the patient in administering a medication are:
   a. oral, sublingual, intravenous injection, and subcutaneous
   b. oral, sublingual, inhalation, and intramuscular injection
   c. absorption, ingestion, inhalation, and exhalation
   d. intramuscular injection, intravenous injection, intraosseous injection, and intradermal injection

2. Before administering or assisting with the administration of a medication:
   a. be sure it was prescribed by a local physician
   b. note what pharmacy the prescription came from
   c. check the medication's expiration date
   d. all of the above

3. The amount of medication to be administered is known as the:
   a. dose
   b. concentration
   c. form
   d. action

4. A situation in which medication should not be administered to a patient because it may cause harm is:
   a. a contraindication
   b. an untoward effect
   c. a dosing regimen
   d. a specification

5. The method by which a medication affects the human body is the:
   a. mode of operation
   b. mechanism of action
   c. symbiotic effect
   d. standard reaction

6. Note "yes" or "no" regarding whether the following medications are normally carried on a BLS EMS unit:
   ___ activated charcoal
   ___ epinephrine
   ___ nitroglycerin
   ___ oral glucose
   ___ oxygen
   ___ prescribed inhaler

7. A side effect is:
   a. an undesirable action of a drug
   b. a life-threatening reaction to a drug
   c. a reason not to administer a drug to a patient
   d. the way a drug affects the body

8. A written protocol or standing order for the use of a medication is an example of:
   a. up-line medical direction
   b. down-line medical direction
   c. off-line medical direction
   d. on-line medical direction

9. Before assisting a patient with taking a prescribed medication, the EMT must be sure the medication was:
   a. prescribed to a family member with a similar problem
   b. purchased at a local pharmacy
   c. prescribed to the patient for the current problem
   d. prescribed by a local doctor

10. After administering a medication, the EMT should note on the run report:
    a. the time the medication was given
    b. the amount of medication given
    c. any response to the medication
    d. all of the above

RESPIRATORY EMERGENCIES

11. Another term for difficulty breathing is:
    a. dysphagia
    b. dissociation
    c. dysrhythmia
    d. dyspnea

12. Signs of difficulty breathing may include all of the following *except:*
    a. wheezing
    b. distended neck veins
    c. an inability to sit upright
    d. extreme anxiety

13. Generally, a patient having difficulty breathing should be given oxygen:
    a. by cannula at 6 lpm
    b. by nonrebreather mask at 15 lpm
    c. only after using a hand-held inhaler
    d. only before using a hand-held inhaler

14. When listening to the lungs of a patient having difficulty breathing, EMTs should be concerned if they hear:
    a. unusual heart sounds
    b. normal breath sounds
    c. wheezing
    d. ascites

15. To make breathing easier, patients having difficulty breathing should be placed:
    a. in a position of comfort
    b. flat on their back
    c. on their left side
    d. in the Trendelenburg position

16. When dealing with a child having breathing problems as opposed to an adult, the EMT must remember:
    a. as long as the child's color is good he or she is getting enough air
    b. retractions are more commonly seen in children than adults
    c. hand-held inhalers should be used only for adults, not children
    d. children seldom experience breathing difficulty as a primary problem

17. The EMT should not assist a patient in using a prescribed inhaler if the patient:
    a. has already used the inhaler once
    b. is wheezing
    c. seems very anxious
    d. has already met the maximum prescribed dose

18. Prior to assisting a patient with a prescribed inhaler:
    a. chill the inhaler in the refrigerator
    b. warm the inhaler in a microwave if one is available
    c. attach the inhaler to an oxygen or compressed air source
    d. shake the inhaler vigorously

19. While depressing the hand-held inhaler, the patient should be instructed to:
    a. inhale deeply
    b. exhale forcefully
    c. swallow
    d. breath normally

20. Immediately after the medication from the inhaler has been delivered, instruct the patient to:
    a. exhale forcefully
    b. cough vigorously
    c. hold his or her breath
    d. swallow

21. A common side effect that may be noted after use of a prescribed inhaler is:
    a. slow pulse
    b. rapid pulse
    c. easier breathing
    d. cyanosis

22. If, after using a prescribed inhaler, the patient has little or no relief, medical direction may instruct the EMT to:
    a. administer a second dose
    b. administer epinephrine
    c. place the patient on oxygen by cannula at 2 lpm
    d. take the patient off oxygen completely

CARDIAC EMERGENCIES

23. The pain commonly associated with cardiac emergencies is usually described as:
    a. a crushing or pressure type of pain
    b. a pain that becomes worse when inhaling deeply
    c. a sharp, stabbing pain
    d. a cramping, intermittent pain

24. Chest pain associated with a cardiac emergency may radiate:
    a. to the jaw
    b. to the shoulder
    c. to either arm
    d. all of the above

✱ 25. A common reaction by a person experiencing chest pain is to:
    a. summon the local EMS
    b. drive to the nearest hospital
    c. deny that he or she may be having a heart problem
    d. immediately call the family doctor

26. A patient experiencing cardiac compromise often:
    a. sweats profusely
    b. feels dry to the touch
    c. is flushed in color
    d. is jaundiced in color

27. Oxygen should be administered to a patient experiencing chest pain:
    a. by cannula at 15 lpm
    b. immediately by nonrebreather mask
    c. only after the EMT has assisted with nitroglycerin
    d. only if the pain is accompanied by difficulty breathing

28. A patient experiencing cardiac compromise should be transported:
    a. lying flat on his or her back
    b. in a prone position
    c. in a position of comfort, preferably semisitting
    d. on his or her left side with the feet slightly elevated

✱ 29. An important aspect of caring for patients with cardiac compromise involves:
    a. telling them they may have died because of waiting to summon help
    b. waiting at the scene to see if oxygen reduces the pain
    c. transporting to their hospital of choice
    d. reassuring them

30. The EMT may assist a patient in taking nitroglycerin if the patient is experiencing:
    a. chest pain and has a history of heart problems
    b. chest pain and there is nitroglycerin in the house
    c. difficulty breathing and dizziness
    d. chest pain associated with difficulty breathing

31. The two common forms of nitroglycerin are:
    a. capsule and tablet
    b. elixir and capsule
    c. tablet and spray
    d. spray and elixir

32. Nitroglycerin works by:
    a. increasing the workload of the heart
    b. dilating the bronchial passages
    c. relaxing the body's blood vessels
    d. constricting the coronary arteries

33. Nitroglycerin should be:
    a. administered under the tongue
    b. swallowed
    c. administered intramuscularly
    d. inhaled

34. Before taking nitroglycerin, the patient's blood pressure must be:
    a. no more than 70 diastolic
    b. at least 80 diastolic
    c. greater than 100 systolic
    d. no more than 120 systolic

35. If a cardiac patient has no relief from pain, medical direction may instruct the EMT to assist with additional doses of nitroglycerin:
    a. every 10 minutes until reaching the hospital
    b. one additional time in 5 minutes
    c. every 8–10 minutes up to a maximum of two doses
    d. every 3–5 minutes up to a maximum of three doses

36. After each dose of nitroglycerin, the EMT should:
    a. reassess the patient's blood pressure
    b. have the patient hold his or her breath
    c. have the patient take a sip of water
    d. check the expiration date of the drug

37. Automated external defibrillation should be performed:
    a. after beginning CPR
    b. immediately after reaching the patient
    c. only if bystander CPR was being performed prior to the EMT's arrival
    d. after placing the patient on oxygen

38. An automated external defibrillator (AED) should *not* be used on patients:
    a. who have drowned
    b. weighing more than 190 pounds
    c. with a known history of cardiac disease
    d. under the age of 12

39. A semiautomated external defibrillator:
    a. advises the EMT whether to administer shock treatments
    b. operates without action on the part of the EMT
    c. uses paddles instead of pads
    d. will automatically deliver an appropriate electrical shock

40. A fully automated external defibrillator:
    a. can be used only on patients weighing less than 150 pounds
    b. operates without action on the part of the EMT, who only needs to turn on the power
    c. can be used by EMTs with no previous training
    d. requires external 110-volt power to operate

41. While the AED is analyzing the patient's cardiac rhythm:
    a. continue CPR
    b. perform ventilations only
    c. discontinue all contact with the patient
    d. check the patient's blood pressure

42. While the AED is delivering a shock:
    a. continue ventilating the patient
    b. do not touch the patient
    c. hold the patient down to prevent jerking and possible injury
    d. continue CPR

43. The patient's pulse should be checked after delivery of:
    a. the first shock only
    b. the second and fourth shock
    c. the third and sixth shock
    d. each shock

44. Between delivery of the first and second series of shocks on a pulseless patient:
    a. do not touch the patient
    b. ventilate the patient only
    c. take the patient's blood pressure
    d. perform CPR for 1 minute

45. If on-scene ALS is not available, the patient should be transported:
    a. after six shocks are delivered
    b. after delivery of the third shock
    c. immediately once the AED indicates that shock is not advisable
    d. prior to attaching the AED

46. If, after delivery of a shock, the patient's pulse returns:
    a. remove the AED from the patient
    b. transport with the AED attached to the patient
    c. continue CPR
    d. continue shocking until six shocks are delivered

47. If a patient needs to be defibrillated in the ambulance:
    a. stop the ambulance prior to defibrillating
    b. continue transporting while defibrillating
    c. stop the ambulance only when the AED is ready to deliver the shock
    d. ground the patient to the vehicle chassis

48. Defibrillation pads should generally be placed:
    a. after CPR is started
    b. over the patient's clothing
    c. on the patient after power is turned on
    d. on the patient before power is turned on

ADDITIONAL POINTS FOR DISCUSSION

Many hospitals now use drugs that can dissolve clots in a coronary artery, restoring blood flow to the heart muscle. These drugs are known as thrombolytics. Early administration of these drugs can make a major difference in patient outcome and quality of life. The EMT is a vital first link in the chain of care for heart attack patients, as the drug must be administered within a certain amount of time after onset of a cardiac emergency. In addition, certain criteria must be met by the patient in order for the drugs to be used.

1. Do any hospitals your department services use these types of drugs?

2. If so, what criteria must a patient meet in order to be considered as a candidate for drug administration?

3. Knowing the criteria and which hospitals may administer the drugs, will this affect:

   * Your patient management?

   * Your decision on where to transport a cardiac emergency patient?

4. Review the operation of your department's AED.

5. Does your department use off-line medical direction, on-line medical direction, or both?

   * What medications can you use with off-line medical direction?

   * What medications can you use with on-line medical direction?

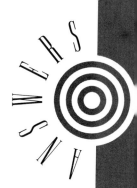

5 MEDICAL EMERGENCIES I

1. b. The routes by which an EMT can administer or assist a patient with administering medications are oral, sublingual, inhalation, and intramuscular injection.

2. c. Before administering or assisting with administering a medication, the EMT should check the medication's expiration date. The pharmacy from where the medication came is not important, nor is it necessary that the medication was prescribed by a local physician.

3. a. The dose is the amount of medication that should be administered to a patient. The correct dose can vary based on the patient's weight and age.

4. a. A contraindication is a situation in which a medication should not be administered to a patient. In such situations, the medication may cause harm or may offer no effect to improve the patient's condition or illness.

5. b. The mechanism of action is the method by which a medication affects the human body.

6. The following medications are normally carried on a BLS EMS unit:
yes activated charcoal
no epinephrine
no nitroglycerin
yes oral glucose
yes oxygen
no prescribed inhaler

7. a. A side effect is an undesirable action of a drug—it is not the same as a contraindication. Side effects may or may not be serious, but they are still unwanted. Knowing the potential side effects of a drug can help prepare the EMT to deal with them if they occur.

8. c. A written protocol or standing order for the use of a medication is an example of off-line medical direction. On-line medical direction refers to a situation where the EMT speaks directly to medical command via a telephone or radio.

9. c. Be sure the medication was prescribed to the patient for the current problem before assisting with its administration. Caution must be exercised because family members often want to be helpful and will give their medication to other family members who appear to have the same problem. The medication does not have to be from a local pharmacy or prescribed by a local doctor as long as it was prescribed for the patient.

10. d. All of the above. Note the time the medication was given, the dose given, and any response (or lack of response) to the medication. Also, note the route by which the medication was administered.

11. d. A patient having difficulty breathing is said to be experiencing dyspnea.

12. c. Patients experiencing difficulty breathing may present sitting upright and leaning forward, or using accessory muscles to try to breathe. Also, wheezing, distended neck veins, extreme anxiety, and bulging eyes may be noted.

13. b. Generally, patients having difficulty breathing should be given oxygen by nonrebreather mask at 15 lpm. Although patients with certain respiratory diseases may develop problems if too much oxygen is given, this is rarely a concern during the short time EMTs treat the patient. EMTs must be careful, however, not to withhold oxygen from a truly hypoxic patient. Remember, if a patient stops breathing because too much oxygen was administered, the EMT can ventilate the patient and sustain life. There are many places worse than the back of an ambulance for this to happen. However, if a patient stops breathing because oxygen was withheld and severe hypoxia developed, the chances of resuscitation are slim.

14. c. The EMT should be concerned if wheezing is heard when listening to a patient's lungs. Note the presence of wheezing on the run sheet and report it to medical command. Ascites is abnormal pooling of fluid in the abdominal cavity.

15. a. To make breathing easier, patients having difficulty breathing should be transported in a position of comfort. Allow the patient to tell you which position makes it easiest to breathe, and try to transport him or her in that position.

16. b. When dealing with children experiencing difficulty breathing, retractions (the use of accessory muscles) are commonly seen (in children more so than adults). In infants, a see-saw breathing pattern, where the abdomen and chest move in opposite directions, may be noted. Don't be fooled if the child's color is good—cyanosis is a late sign of breathing distress in children.

17. d. If the patient has used an inhaler prior to the arrival of EMS and has reached the maximum prescribed dose, do not give additional medication. Patients having difficulty breathing may present with wheezing and anxiety, both of which may be alleviated after taking medication.

18. d. Shake the inhaler vigorously several times prior to administering the medication. Although the inhaler should be at room temperature, do not use a microwave to warm it. Inhalers are already under pressure and do not need external compressed gas sources for power.

19. a. To deliver the medication, instruct the patient to inhale deeply while depressing the handheld inhaler.

20. c. Immediately after inhaling the medication, have the patient hold his or her breath for as long as is comfortably possible. This will allow the medication to be absorbed.

21. b. After using the prescribed inhaler, the patient may experience a rapid pulse; however, this is usually not of great concern. If the medication does its job, the patient should experience some relief from the difficulty breathing.

22. a. If the first dose does not produce the desired results, medical direction may authorize a second dose. Oxygen is still of critical importance, as the patient's blood oxygen level may have dropped markedly during the episode. It is most appropriately administered to the patient via a nonrebreather mask.

23. a. A crushing pain or heavy pressure that radiates into other parts of the body is most often associated with a cardiac emergency. The pain is seldom described as sharp or stabbing and is usually not affected by inhaling deeply.

24. **d.** All of the above. Chest pain most commonly radiates to the left arm, but may radiate to either arm, the jaw, either shoulder, the back, or the abdomen.

25. **c.** People having chest pain commonly deny that they are having heart problems such as a heart attack. These patients will wait an average of 3 hours before calling for help.

26. **a.** A patient experiencing a cardiac emergency often sweats profusely (is diaphoretic) and is pale.

27. **b.** Oxygen should immediately be administered by nonrebreather mask at 15 lpm to the cardiac emergency patient. A lack of oxygen to the heart muscle can cause permanent damage and death.

28. **c.** Patients experiencing cardiac compromise should be transported in a position of comfort. Usually, they are most comfortable in a semisitting position.

29. **d.** The patient should be constantly reassured. He or she may now realize the seriousness of the situation and start to worry about death. Do not ridicule or counsel the patient. To reduce the risk of sudden death from an abnormal cardiac rhythm, the patient should be transported to the closest hospital.

30. **a.** If a patient is experiencing chest pain, has a history of heart problems, and has a personal prescription for nitroglycerin, the EMT may receive permission to assist the patient in taking the medication.

31. **c.** The nitroglycerin an EMT may assist in administering is commonly prescribed in a tablet or spray form.

32. **c.** Nitroglycerin relaxes the body's blood vessels, thereby decreasing the workload of the heart.

33. **a.** Regardless of whether the medication is in tablet or spray form, nitroglycerin is administered sublingually, that is, under the patient's tongue. Make sure the patient understands this. Although the medication was prescribed to the patient, some do not understand that the medication should not be swallowed or chewed. Nitroglycerin spray should not be inhaled.

34. **c.** The patient's blood pressure must be greater than 100 systolic before nitroglycerin is given.

35. **d.** If the pain is not relieved, the EMT may be permitted to give nitroglycerin every 3–5 minutes for a total of three doses (including the initial dose).

36. **a.** Reassess the patient's blood pressure after each dose of nitroglycerin. This should be performed about 2 minutes after the patient takes the medication.

37. **b.** If an automated external defibrillator (AED) is available on the scene, automated external defibrillation should be performed immediately after reaching the patient, even before starting CPR.

38. **d.** An AED should not be used on patients younger than 12 years or weighing less than 90 pounds.

39. **a.** A semiautomated external defibrillator advises the EMT whether to administer electrical shocks. The EMT must then activate the shock. This means that there is a risk of not delivering an appropriate shock if the EMT does not activate the unit.

40. **b.** A fully automated external defibrillator operates with no action on the part of the EMT other than to turn on the power. All AEDs carried on ambulances are capable of battery operation. EMTs still need to be trained in the proper use of an AED.

41. **c.** While the AED is analyzing the patient's cardiac rhythm, EMTs should discontinue all contact with the patient, including CPR. This allows the unit to properly analyze the cardiac rhythm.

42. **b.** While an automated external defibrillator is delivering a shock, EMTs should not touch the patient. There is a risk of accidental shock to the rescuers if they come in contact with the patient.

43. **c.** Shocks are delivered in series of three. Check the patient's pulse after the third and sixth shock.

44. **d.** If the first series of shocks does not convert the patient to a normal rhythm, perform CPR for 1 minute, then deliver the second series of shocks.

45. **a.** If on-scene ALS is not available, it is generally recommended that the EMT transport the patient after six shocks are delivered or the AED gives three consecutive messages (separated by 1 minute of CPR) that a shock is not advised. Because guidelines regarding when to transport the patient may vary from area to area, local protocols should be followed.

46. **b.** If the patient's pulse returns after delivery of a shock, discontinue CPR, load the patient, and transport. Because the patient may go into cardiac arrest again, leave the AED attached to the patient but turned off (if it is a fully automatic model).

47. **a.** Stop the ambulance before attempting defibrillation. Although defibrillation can be performed in an ambulance, the AED cannot adequately analyze the patient's cardiac rhythm in a bouncing vehicle. Also, there is more risk of an EMT being accidently shocked in a moving ambulance.

48. **d.** Generally, defibrillator pads should be placed on the patient and connected to the AED before the EMT turns on the power. Consult the manufacturer's instructions for exact guidelines. Defibrillator pads must be placed directly on the skin.

CHAPTER 6

MEDICAL EMERGENCIES II

ALTERED MENTAL STATUS

1. Common causes of altered mental status include:
   a. poisoning
   b. infection
   c. decreased oxygen levels
   d. all of the above

2. The first priority in managing a patient with altered mental status is:
   a. administering sugar
   b. assuring an adequate airway
   c. performing a focused exam
   d. assessing baseline vitals

3. Of particular importance to the EMT who has encountered a patient with altered mental status is:
   a. the age and weight of the patient
   b. a detailed assessment
   c. patient history
   d. whether the patient has a prescribed inhaler

4. Diabetes is a condition in which:
   a. there is not enough sugar in the bloodstream
   b. the body is unable to utilize sugar normally
   c. insulin is overproduced
   d. the cells produce too much sugar

5. Hypoglycemia is characterized by:
   a. low blood sugar
   b. high blood sugar
   c. not enough insulin
   d. slow metabolism

6. A hypoglycemic patient may:
   a. appear intoxicated
   b. have flushed skin
   c. have a slow pulse
   d. present with dry skin

7. Two questions that should be asked of a diabetic patient are:
   a. "Have you eaten today?" and "Do you know where you are?"
   b. "Have you eaten today?" and "Have you taken your medication today?"
   c. "Do you know where you are?" and "What day is today?"
   d. "Have you taken your medication today?" and "What day is today?"

8. A medication commonly taken by diabetic patients is:
   a. nitroglycerine
   b. antihistamines
   c. aspirin
   d. insulin

9. Hypoglycemia may be caused by:
   a. an unusually strenuous exercise or physical work episode
   b. eating too much
   c. taking too little insulin
   d. all of the above

10. Oral glucose should be given to a patient with altered mental status and a:
    a. history of heart problems
    b. history of diabetes
    c. recent head injury
    d. recent episode of difficulty breathing

11. Oral glucose comes in the form of a:
    a. liquid suspension
    b. powder
    c. gel
    d. tablet

12. Oral glucose should not be given to patients who:
    a. already drank a sugar-containing solution
    b. are unable to protect their airway
    c. have vomited
    d. are responsive

13. The normal initial dose of oral glucose is:
    a. ¼ tube
    b. ½ tube
    c. 1 tube
    d. 2 tubes

14. Oral glucose should be placed:
    a. on the patient's tongue
    b. between the patient's cheek and gums
    c. at the back of the patient's throat
    d. on the patient's teeth

15. The greatest danger associated with use of oral glucose is:
    a. allergic reactions
    b. side effects
    c. sugar overload
    d. aspiration

SEIZURES

16. A patient who experiences a seizure has:
    a. diabetes
    b. violent muscular activity
    c. status epilepticus
    d. abnormal electric activity in the brain

17. Concerning seizures, the EMT must remember that:
    a. they are always life-threatening
    b. they signify that the patient has epilepsy
    c. there are many causes
    d. there is always an associated medical history

18. In children, a seizure that is associated with a high temperature is known as:
    a. focal
    b. febrile
    c. hypothermic
    d. petit mal

19. EMTs should be aware that seizures may be caused by:
    a. increased levels of oxygen
    b. head trauma
    c. psychotic behavior
    d. all of the above

✳ 20. The movement associated with a seizure:
    a. may range from violent jerking to simple staring episodes
    b. always affects the entire body
    c. generally starts in one area then moves to another
    d. demonstrates combative behavior on the part of the patient

✳ 21. The EMT should be particularly concerned if a patient experiences:
    a. the same type of seizure that he or she has had in the past
    b. repeated, uncontrolled seizures with no return of consciousness between episodes
    c. a seizure involving one limb
    d. a full-body seizure with no loss of consciousness

✱ 22. When managing a patient who is actively seizing:
   a. physically restrain the patient
   b. protect the patient from further injury
   c. force a bite stick between the patient's front teeth
   d. administer glucose under the tongue

23. During the period immediately following a generalized seizure, the patient is likely to be:
   a. alert and oriented to place and time
   b. sleepy but aware of what has happened
   c. unresponsive or difficult to arouse
   d. hyperactive and unable to stay still

24. After a patient has experienced a seizure and if there is no associated cervical spine trauma, the patient should be positioned:
   a. prone
   b. supine
   c. in the shock position
   d. in the recovery position

✱ 25. If an adult patient with a history of seizures has experienced a seizure, is now alert and oriented, but does not want to go to the hospital, the EMT should:
   a. restrain the patient and take him or her to the hospital
   b. thoroughly document the incident and allow the patient to sign a refusal form
   c. have the patient take an extra dose of antiseizure medication
   d. ridicule the patient for not going to the hospital

ALLERGIC REACTIONS

26. An allergic reaction may include:
   a. hives and itching
   b. difficulty breathing
   c. a tight feeling in the throat
   d. all of the above

27. The most common complication of a serious allergic reaction is:
   a. hypoperfusion
   b. slow heart rate
   c. difficulty breathing
   d. increased blood pressure

28. Concerning allergic reactions, it must be remembered that:
   a. the reaction may affect many parts of the body
   b. all reactions occur to the same extent
   c. all patients react in the same way to an allergen
   d. the reaction is limited to the immediate area of the exposure to the allergen

29. Unlike other forms of breathing problems, the difficulty breathing that is experienced by a patient having an allergic reaction may be caused by:
   a. widespread dilation of the bronchial passages
   b. swelling of the neck and respiratory tract
   c. bacteria in the throat
   d. inability of the diaphragm to contract

30. The altered mental status exhibited by some patients having a severe allergic reaction is due to:
   a. constriction of blood vessels in the brain
   b. increased blood pressure
   c. low blood sugar
   d. hypoperfusion

31. The use of epinephrine is indicated:
   a. if a patient is having an allergic reaction accompanied by difficulty breathing or hypoperfusion
   b. for any patient experiencing an allergic reaction
   c. if a patient is having an allergic reaction accompanied by hives and itching
   d. for any patient with an epinephrine prescription who has been stung by a bee

32. The effects of epinephrine on the respiratory and circulatory systems include:
   a. dilating bronchioles and blood vessels
   b. constricting bronchioles and dilating blood vessels
   c. dilating bronchioles and constricting blood vessels
   d. constricting bronchioles and blood vessels

33. A contraindication for using epinephrine when a person is experiencing a severe allergic reaction is:
   a. hypersensitivity to bee stings
   b. a history of asthma
   c. a patient younger than 16 years
   d. there is no contraindication

34. Epinephrine used to manage an allergic reaction is administered:
   a. intravenously
   b. intramuscularly
   c. subcutaneously
   d. intradermally

35. The adult dose of epinephrine for an allergic reaction is:
   a. 0.1 mg
   b. 0.2 mg
   c. 0.3 mg
   d. 0.4 mg

36. The dose of epinephrine for infants or children experiencing an allergic reaction is:
   a. 0.05 mg
   b. 0.15 mg
   c. 0.25 mg
   d. 0.35 mg

37. The preferred anatomic location for administering epinephrine is:
   a. the lateral portion of the thigh, midway between the waist and the knee
   b. the buttocks
   c. the abdomen, immediately below the navel
   d. the medial portion of the forearm, midway between the elbow and the wrist

38. In order for the autoinjector to work:
   a. it is preferable but not always necessary to remove the clothing over the injection site
   b. the clothing must be removed over the injection site
   c. the injector must be filled by the EMT
   d. a needle must be attached to the injector by the EMT

39. After the injector activates:
   a. remove it immediately
   b. move it to an alternate spot and activate it again
   c. reset it for use on the next patient
   d. hold it in place for 10 seconds

40. Side effects of epinephrine include:
   a. decreased pulse rate and pale skin
   b. decreased pulse rate and flushed skin
   c. increased pulse rate and flushed skin
   d. increased pulse rate and pale skin

41. If a patient's condition continues to deteriorate after epinephrine is administered:
   a. the patient is most likely experiencing a reaction to the epinephrine itself
   b. half the original dose should be administered
   c. an additional dose may be ordered
   d. defibrillate the patient using an AED.

ADDITIONAL POINTS FOR DISCUSSION

1. What brand or brands of oral glucose are carried on your ambulance? Review the directions for administration.

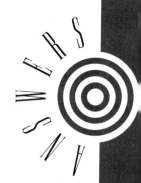

6 MEDICAL EMERGENCIES II

1. **d.** All of the above. Altered mental status may be caused by poisoning, infection, or decreased oxygen levels. It may also be caused by head trauma or hypoglycemia or may be noted after a seizure.

2. **b.** Assuring an adequate airway is the first concern during management of a patient with altered mental status.

3. **c.** The patient history is of particular importance when a patient with altered mental status is encountered. The history enables the EMT to determine whether the condition is related to an ongoing medical problem or is a new occurrence.

4. **b.** Diabetes is a condition in which the body is unable to utilize sugar normally.

5. **a.** Hypoglycemia is characterized by low blood sugar.

6. **a.** A hypoglycemic patient may seem intoxicated. Because of this, the EMT must use caution when assessing a patient who is believed to be drunk—misdiagnosis could be deadly. The hypoglycemic patient normally presents with pale, moist skin, and a rapid pulse.

7. **b.** Diabetic patients should be asked if they have eaten today and taken their medication today. If the patient is unconscious, ask a family member these questions.

8. **d.** Diabetic patients may take insulin. Insulin allows glucose to cross the cell membrane.

9. **a.** Hypoglycemia may occur after an unusually strenuous exercise or physical work episode. It may also occur if the patient eats too little or vomits after eating, or if the patient has taken too much insulin.

10. **b.** A patient with altered mental status and a history of diabetes should be given oral glucose.

11. **c.** Oral glucose comes in the form of a gel.

12. **b.** Oral glucose should not be given to someone who is unable to protect his or her airway. It should not be given to unconscious patients or those who are unable to swallow.

13. **c.** The normal initial dose of oral glucose is 1 tube.

14. **b.** Oral glucose should be placed between the patient's cheek and gums.

15. **d.** The greatest danger associated with use of oral glucose is aspiration into the lungs.

16. d. Abnormal electric activity in the brain is associated with seizures. Not all patients with seizures have epilepsy, and seizures do not always involve muscular activity.

17. c. There are many causes of seizures. Seizures normally are not life-threatening although they can be frightening. The patient does not always have an associated medical history or epilepsy.

18. b. A febrile seizure is a seizure associated with a high temperature, and is normally seen in infants and children.

19. b. When a patient has experienced head trauma, a seizure may occur.

20. a. Seizures may be characterized by violent jerking of parts of the body or may be as simple as a staring episode. The EMT should carefully note on the run report the area of the body involved and how it was affected.

21. b. Repeated, uncontrolled seizures with no return of consciousness between episodes is a true emergency.

22. b. An EMT should protect an actively seizing patient from further injury and, if possible, from embarrassment. The only time a patient should be physically restrained is if the patient is in danger of physically harming himself or herself. Bite blocks are not recommended in most areas; however, if they are used, they should not be placed while the patient is actively seizing. If called for by local protocol, bite blocks should be placed between the molars. Do not put glucose in the patient's mouth, as it may be aspirated into the lungs.

23. c. During the period immediately following a generalized seizure, the patient is most likely to be unresponsive or difficult to arouse. This is known as the postictal phase or period. As time passes, the patient will become more oriented to person, place, and time, but may not remember having a seizure.

24. d. After a patient has experienced a seizure, he or she should be placed in the recovery position if there is no associated cervical spine trauma.

25. b. An adult patient with a history of seizures who is alert and oriented has the right to refuse transport, even if he or she has recently had a seizure. The EMTs should thoroughly document the incident and explain to the patient their concern about not transporting and their willingness to do so. If he or she still does not want to go, have the patient sign a refusal.

26. d. All of the above. Signs and symptoms of an allergic reaction may include itching and hives, difficulty breathing, and a tight feeling in the throat. Also, wheezing, increased heart rate, decreased blood pressure, and a variety of other signs and symptoms may be noted.

27. c. Difficulty breathing is the most common complication of an allergic reaction. The patient may also experience severe hypoperfusion and eventual death.

28. a. Although the allergic reaction may result from some local event, such as a bite or a sting, the reaction may affect other parts of the body. Reactions can vary, depending on the patient.

29. **b.** The difficulty breathing experienced by a person having an allergic reaction may be related to swelling of the neck and respiratory tract.

30. **d.** The altered mental status exhibited by some patients having a severe allergic reaction is due to hypoperfusion.

31. **a.** Epinephrine should be administered to a patient who has been prescribed the medication and is experiencing an allergic reaction accompanied by difficulty breathing or hypoperfusion. Use of the drug is not indicated simply because the patient has been stung by a bee or is experiencing a mild allergic reaction.

32. **c.** Epinephrine dilates bronchioles and constricts blood vessels. Bronchiole dilatation enables the patient to breathe easier, and blood vessel constriction increases blood pressure, thereby improving perfusion to the brain.

33. **d.** There is no contraindication for using epinephrine when a person is experiencing a severe allergic reaction. Epinephrine can even be used in infants and children.

34. **b.** Epinephrine used to manage an allergic reaction is injected intramuscularly.

35. **c.** The adult dose of epinephrine for an allergic reaction is 0.3 mg.

36. **b.** The dose of epinephrine for infants and children experiencing an allergic reaction is 0.15 mg.

37. **a.** The preferred location for administering epinephrine is the lateral portion of the thigh, midway between the waist and the knee. Some areas allow the fleshy portion of the upper arm to be used also. Consult your local protocols.

38. **a.** In order for the autoinjector to work, it is preferable to remove the clothing over the site. However, if clothing is thin enough, the injection can be performed through it. The injector comes prefilled with the medication and with the needle attached.

39. **d.** After the injector activates, hold it in place for 10 seconds to allow the medication to be injected. Dispose of the autoinjector in an approved container for sharp instruments.

40. **d.** Side effects of epinephrine include an increased pulse rate and pale skin. The patient may also complain of dizziness, chest pain, headache, and may become nauseated and vomit.

41. **c.** If a patient's condition continues to deteriorate after epinephrine is administered, an additional dose may be ordered by medical control.

CHAPTER 7

POISONING/OVERDOSE AND ENVIRONMENTAL EMERGENCIES

POISONING/OVERDOSE

1. Four main ways poison enters the body are:
   a. injection, inhalation, ingestion, and insect stings
   b. unintentional, absorption, accidental, and intentional
   c. ingestion, inhalation, injection, and absorption
   d. direct, inhalation, indirect, and ingestion

2. Most poisonings in children are related to:
   a. drug abuse
   b. surface contact
   c. accidental ingestion
   d. child abuse

3. Accidental poisoning should be suspected if a patient displays:
   a. discoloration around the mouth and lips
   b. burning or pain in the mouth, throat, or stomach
   c. difficulty talking or swallowing
   d. all of the above

4. With orders from medical direction, management of a patient who has ingested poison may include:
   a. degrading the poison
   b. making the patient vomit
   c. attempting to locate a specific antidote for the poison
   d. administering activated charcoal

5. An important factor when managing a poisoning patient that is less critical for other emergency patients is the patient's:
   a. date of birth
   b. weight
   c. medical history
   d. allergy history

6. Any containers, bottles, or labels that are found at the scene of a poisoning emergency should be:
   a. taken to the receiving hospital
   b. given to a hazardous materials team
   c. given to law enforcement officers
   d. destroyed immediately to prevent contamination of personnel

7. When a person who has ingested poison is encountered, the EMT should try to determine:
   a. what the substance tasted like
   b. how much of the substance was ingested
   c. where the substance was obtained
   d. how old the substance is

8. The EMT should attempt to determine exactly when a substance was ingested because:
   a. the information may affect management of the patient
   b. many substances lose their potency after a certain period
   c. if no ill effects are noted after 2 or 3 hours, the patient probably is not in danger
   d. antidotes administered at the hospital must be given within 1 hour of ingestion

9. Ingested poisons may particularly affect the:
   a. respiratory tract
   b. cardiovascular system
   c. gastrointestinal tract
   d. nervous system

10. A major concern when dealing with inhaled poisons is that they:
    a. all may be exhaled by the patient and contaminate the EMT
    b. may also damage the lining of the patient's airway
    c. take longer to enter the blood stream
    d. all of the above

11. The first step in managing a victim who has inhaled poison gas is to:
    a. apply oxygen
    b. determine the type of gas involved
    c. open the airway and assess breathing
    d. remove the patient from the toxic environment

12. An early sign of carbon monoxide poisoning is:
    a. cherry-red color of the skin
    b. headache, nausea, and vomiting
    c. unconsciousness
    d. chest pain radiating to the left arm

13. During an incident involving poison gas, the EMT must remember that:
    a. poison gases have distinct odors that make them readily identifiable
    b. poison gases are lighter than air and rapidly dissipate
    c. the poison gas may still be present but undetectable by the EMT
    d. the patient will improve once he or she is out of the toxic environment

14. Insect and spider bites are examples of poisons that enter the body through:
    a. absorption
    b. subjection
    c. trajection
    d. injection

15. If poisoning was caused by an animal:
    a. be careful not to become a victim also
    b. take whatever means necessary to catch the animal for identification
    c. transport the patient to a rabies control center
    d. do not be concerned because animal bites are cleaner than human bites

16. Dry fertilizer is an example of a poison that enters the body through:
    a. injection
    b. absorption
    c. osmosis
    d. digestion

17. Management of a patient who has been poisoned by contact with a powdered chemical would include:
    a. brushing off or washing off any chemical
    b. leaving the chemical in place so it can be later identified
    c. diluting the chemical with a light mist of water
    d. wrapping the patient in a sheet to prevent spreading of the chemical

18. When liquid toxins are encountered on the skin, the site should be irrigated:
    a. with sterile water
    b. until an odor is no longer present
    c. for at least 20 minutes
    d. until the site looks clean

19. If a child has handled or been poisoned by a corrosive substance, the EMT should:
    a. wash the child's hands and fingers
    b. administer syrup of ipecac
    c. bandage the hands
    d. wear rubber gloves and a mask

20. Activated charcoal may be useful in managing poisons that enter the body:
    a. intravenously
    b. through the lungs
    c. over a prolonged period
    d. through ingestion

21. Activated charcoal is useful in cases involving poisonings because it:
    a. causes vomiting
    b. decreases stomach motility
    c. prevents the body from absorbing a poison
    d. is a direct antidote for most poisons

22. Activated charcoal used by EMTs is normally:
    a. a powder
    b. a gel
    c. a tablet
    d. premixed in water

23. Contraindications for using activated charcoal include all of the following *except:*
    a. inability to swallow
    b. ingestion of detergents
    c. altered mental status
    d. ingestion of acids and alkalis

24. The usual adult dose for activated charcoal is:
    a. 5–12.5 grams
    b. 12.5–25 grams
    c. 25–50 grams
    d. 50–75 grams

25. The usual dose of activated charcoal for infants and children is:
    a. 5–12.5 grams
    b. 12.5–25 grams
    c. 25–50 grams
    d. 50–75 grams

26. When basing the dose of activated charcoal on a patient's weight, the dose is:
    a. 1 g/kg for both children and adults
    b. 1 g/kg for adults and 0.5 g/kg for children
    c. 0.5 g/kg for both children and adults
    d. 2 g/kg for adults and 1 g/kg for children

27. Before administering activated charcoal:
    a. shake the container vigorously
    b. mix the charcoal with water
    c. avoid agitating the container
    d. tell the patient it tastes good

28. A normal side effect that may be associated with activated charcoal is:
    a. diarrhea
    b. abdominal cramps
    c. heartburn
    d. black stools

29. If the patient vomits shortly after taking activated charcoal:
    a. repeat the activated charcoal at twice the initial dose
    b. administer syrup of ipecac
    c. repeat the dose one time
    d. do not give any more activated charcoal

ENVIRONMENTAL EMERGENCIES

30. A direct transfer of heat from a warm body to a cooler object, such as if a person were immersed in cold water, is:
    a. conduction
    b. evaporation
    c. convection
    d. radiation

31. A medical condition that could predispose a patient to hypothermia is:
    a. asthma
    b. obesity
    c. spinal injury
    d. high blood pressure

32. Infants and young children are more at risk than adults for hypothermia because they:
    a. have a smaller body surface area
    b. have more body fat
    c. have slower pulse rates
    d. do not shiver as efficiently

33. To assess a suspected hypothermia patient's body temperature, feel the patient's:
    a. abdominal skin
    b. forehead
    c. arms
    d. feet

34. When a patient becomes hypothermic, shivering:
    a. is always present
    b. is not present
    c. may or may not be present
    d. is undesirable

35. In the early stages of hypothermia, a patient's vital signs typically include a:
    a. rapid pulse rate and slow breathing
    b. slow pulse rate and rapid breathing
    c. slow pulse rate and slow breathing
    d. rapid pulse rate and rapid breathing

36. During management of a hypothermic patient, alcoholic beverages should:
    a. be given if available
    b. be given only if the patient has no history of alcoholism
    c. never be given
    d. be warmed before being given to the patient

37. Management of a hypothermic patient who is alert and responding appropriately would include:
    a. having the patient walk vigorously
    b. rewarming the patient by applying heat packs to the groin, armpits, and neck areas
    c. massaging arms and legs to stimulate circulation
    d. giving the patient hot coffee to drink

38. When dealing with a severely hypothermic, unresponsive patient:
    a. hyperventilate the patient
    b. do not perform external cardiac massage, as it may cause ventricular fibrillation
    c. handle the patient very gently, avoiding rough movements
    d. do not administer oxygen

39. Before beginning CPR on an unresponsive hypothermia patient, check the:
    a. radial pulse for 20 seconds
    b. radial pulse for 1 minute
    c. carotid pulse for 15 seconds
    d. carotid pulse for 30–45 seconds

✴ 40. A good guideline to follow when dealing with an unresponsive hypothermia patient is:
    a. resuscitation should only be attempted on a patient who has been hypothermic less than 20 minutes
    b. the patient is not dead until he or she is warm and dead
    c. a patient with muscle rigidity should not be resuscitated
    d. if the patient appears dead, he or she is probably dead

41. A superficial local cold-related injury is characterized by:
    a. blanching of the skin
    b. white, waxy skin
    c. frozen feeling upon palpation
    d. blisters

42. A sign of a deep local cold-related injury is:
    a. soft skin
    b. moist skin
    c. white, waxy skin
    d. tingling in the injured area

43. If an early or superficial local cold-related injury is noted on an extremity:
    a. splint the extremity
    b. rub or massage the affected area
    c. apply snow to the area if available
    d. leave the area uncovered

44. To manage a late or deep cold-related injury:
    a. apply heat to the area
    b. break any blister that may have formed to allow cold fluid to escape
    c. cover the area with dry dressings
    d. rub or massage the affected area to restore circulation

45. A local cold-related injury may need to be rewarmed if:
    a. the patient develops severe pain
    b. extremely long or delayed transport is inevitable
    c. the area is likely to refreeze
    d. the patient is unresponsive

46. If it is necessary to rewarm a local cold-related injury in the field, it should be accomplished:
    a. gradually in cool water
    b. rapidly in very hot water
    c. gradually using rubbing alcohol
    d. rapidly in warm water

47. When dressing hands or feet after rewarming:
    a. place dry, sterile dressings between the fingers or toes
    b. use an occlusive dressing
    c. use moist dressings
    d. wrap them tightly using elastic bandages

48. Climate contributes to the chances of heat-related emergencies if:
    a. barometric pressure is low
    b. there is high relative humidity
    c. it is warm and dry
    d. ambient temperature is low

49. Elderly patients are at particular risk for heat-related emergencies because they:
    a. are very mobile and cannot remove their own clothing
    b. have higher pulse rates and low blood pressure
    c. are less sensitive to heat and have better blood supply to the extremities
    d. have poor thermoregulation and may take many medications

50. After ensuring an adequate airway, the first step in managing the victim of a heat-related emergency is to:
    a. remove the patient from the hot environment
    b. lay the patient on the left side
    c. loosen the patient's clothing
    d. drench the patient with cold water

51. The muscle cramps that may accompany a heat-related emergency are believed to be related to:
    a. excessive blood supply to the muscles
    b. a loss of body salts
    c. hypothermia
    d. heat exhaustion

52. A dire emergency exists if a patient has:
    a. moist, pale, normal temperature skin
    b. moist, pale, cool temperature skin
    c. moist, pink, normal temperature skin
    d. dry or moist, hot temperature skin

53. Heat-related emergency patients should be given water to drink if they are:
    a. feeling nauseated
    b. semiresponsive and have dry, hot skin
    c. responsive and have moist, pale, normal to cool temperature skin
    d. complaining of thirst

54. An important early step in managing a patient with skin that is hot to the touch is to:
    a. conserve body heat to prevent rebound hypothermia
    b. wipe down the patient with rubbing alcohol
    c. keep the skin dry
    d. apply cold packs to the neck, groin, and armpits

55. The difference between near-drowning and drowning is:
    a. near-drowning occurs close to shore
    b. near-drowning does not involve aspiration of water into the lungs
    c. near-drowning patients survive at least temporarily after the incident
    d. near-drowning patients have not stopped breathing

56. Early management of a drowning or near-drowning patient primarily involves:
    a. caring for hypovolemic shock
    b. early respiratory and circulatory support
    c. removing water from the lungs
    d. reversing acidosis

57. Any patient found unconscious in a swimming pool should be suspected of having:
    a. spinal injuries
    b. a heart attack
    c. abdominal injuries
    d. rib fractures

✱ 58. When rescuing an unconscious patient from a swimming pool:
    a. wait until the patient is out of the water to start artificial ventilation
    b. move the patient to the side of the pool in the position found
    c. start chest compressions while the patient is still in the water if there is no pulse
    d. roll the patient face up as soon as possible while providing spinal support

59. A cold water, near-drowning patient:
    a. should not be resuscitated if submerged longer than 30 minutes
    b. should be aggressively rewarmed in the back of the ambulance
    c. may survive even after a long submersion time
    d. is likely to have brain damage if resuscitated

60. If spinal injury is not suspected, a breathing, near-drowning patient should be placed:
    a. on the left side
    b. in a prone position
    c. in the shock position
    d. in the Trendelenburg position

61. If gastric distention interferes with artificial ventilation on a drowning patient, the EMT should:
    a. discontinue ventilations and perform chest compressions only
    b. place the patient on his or her left side and apply firm pressure over the epigastric area
    c. use more forceful ventilations
    d. insert a suction catheter as far as possible into the patient's throat to remove stomach contents

62. When removing a stinger, the EMT should:
    a. scrape it off
    b. grasp it with a pair of tweezers and pull gently
    c. freeze the stinger with an ice cube before removing
    d. coat the stinger with petroleum jelly before removing

63. If possible, the injection site of a sting or bite should be:
    a. elevated above the level of the patient's heart
    b. massaged gently during transport
    c. directly rubbed with ice
    d. slightly below the level of the patient's heart

64. When managing a snakebite victim:
    a. apply heat to the bite area
    b. do not apply cold to the bite area
    c. elevate the bite area if an extremity is involved
    d. try to keep the patient active

65. If a snakebite is encountered, a constricting band should be used:
    a. on all pit viper bites
    b. only if the snake can be immediately captured
    c. only after consulting medical direction
    d. if incision and suction are to be performed

66. While managing a patient with a sting or bite, the EMT should be alert for the potential development of:
a. low blood sugar
b. cellulitis
c. an allergic reaction
d. high blood pressure

ADDITIONAL POINTS FOR DISCUSSION

1. What is the phone number of your local poison control center?

2. What are your local protocols regarding rewarming of:

  * Hypothermia patients?

  * Local cold injuries?

3. What venomous animals or insects are common in your area? *Note:* Many may be found in private collections, not just in the wild.

4. What medical facilities in your area are best suited to treat poisonous animal bites or stings?

5. There is no universal snake antivenin. The snake must be identified, and the specific type of antivenin administered. If a poisonous snakebite is encountered:

  * How would you go about getting a positive identification of the type of snake involved?

  * Where is the closest supply of snake antivenin located, and what specific snakebites can be treated?

6. What are your local protocols regarding management of:

  * Poisonous snakebites?

  * Marine life stings?

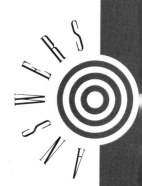
7 POISONING/OVERDOSE AND ENVIRONMENTAL EMERGENCIES

1. **c.** The four main ways poison enters the body are through ingestion, inhalation, injection, and absorption.

2. **c.** Accidental ingestion accounts for most poisonings in children.

3. **d.** All of the above. If a patient displays discoloration around the mouth and lips; has burning or pain in the mouth, throat, or stomach; or has difficulty talking or swallowing, suspect poisoning.

4. **d.** With orders from medical command, the EMT may administer activated charcoal to some poisoning patients. Inducing vomiting in the field is no longer indicated. Do not waste time trying to locate a specific antidote for the poison.

5. **b.** The weight of a patient is of particular concern when managing a poisoning patient. The same amount of poison will have greater effects on a person with less body weight than a person with greater body weight.

6. **a.** Any containers, bottles, or labels that are found at the scene of a poisoning emergency should be taken to the receiving hospital. Take care, however, not to contaminate medical personnel or equipment when collecting or transporting the substance or container.

7. **b.** If possible, try to determine how much of a substance was ingested because the information can affect treatment. This may not always be easy if the poisoning involves a small child or if a patient has accidently ingested poison.

8. **a.** Although finding a specific antidote is not important, trying to determine when a poison was ingested is, as this may affect management of the patient. The effects of some poisons may not be noted for several hours after exposure.

9. **c.** Ingested poisons may particularly affect the gastrointestinal tract. The patient may experience nausea, vomiting, abdominal cramps, and diarrhea.

10. **b.** Inhaled poisons may also damage the lining of the patient's airway. In general, these poisons are rapidly absorbed into the bloodstream through the capillaries in the lungs. There usually is no danger that the EMT will be poisoned by the patient's exhaled air. However, solvents inhaled to get high may be excreted by the lungs and pose a danger to a rescuer doing mouth-to-mouth resuscitation.

11. **d.** Before all else, remove poison gas victims from the toxic environment. This should only be done while wearing protective equipment, such as a self-contained breathing apparatus.

12. b. Headache, nausea, and vomiting are early signs of carbon monoxide poisoning. The headache is caused by widespread dilatation of the cerebral arteries. A cherry-red color of the skin is a late sign of poisoning.

13. c. Caution must be exercised during incidents involving poison gas because the gas may still be present but undetectable by the EMTs. Some gases have no odor, color, or taste. The patient's condition may continue to deteriorate even after removal from the toxic environment because the poison is already in the patient's bloodstream.

14. d. The poison from insect and spider bites enters the body by injection.

15. a. Because EMTs may not be familiar with methods of handling poisonous insects or animals, be careful not to become a victim also. The capture and identification of such animals should be performed by qualified personnel.

16. b. Dry fertilizer is a poison that enters the body through absorption.

17. a. Chemicals that have contacted the body should be brushed off if dry, or washed off if liquid. The chemical must be removed to decrease further absorption.

18. c. When a patient is contaminated by a liquid toxin, irrigate the contaminated area for at least 20 minutes. Rather than delay transport, irrigation can normally be accomplished enroute to the hospital. The water should be clean but does not have to be sterile. Just because the site looks clean or an odor is no longer present does not mean that all the toxin has been removed.

19. a. Wash the hands and fingers of a child who has handled or been poisoned by corrosives. This prevents eye damage that may be caused if the child rubs his or her eyes. Wearing rubber gloves may be indicated, but a mask is not necessary and may upset the child. Be careful to avoid being splattered while cleaning the child.

20. d. Activated charcoal is used to treat patients who have ingested certain poisons. Poisons that enter the body over a long period, regardless of the method of entry, tend to be more difficult to treat.

21. c. Activated charcoal prevents the poison from being absorbed into the body through the gastrointestinal tract. It works by adsorbing (not absorbing) poisons, that is, it binds with the toxins. This allows them to pass through the system causing minimal harm.

22. d. The activated charcoal used by EMTs comes premixed in water. Although it is available as a powder, this form is not recommended for use in the field.

23. b. Contraindications for the use of activated charcoal include inability to swallow, altered mental status, and ingestion of acids and alkalis.

24. c. The usual adult dose of activated charcoal is 25–50 grams.

25. b. The usual dose of activated charcoal for infants and children is 12.5–25 grams, approximately one-half the adult dose.

26. a. When using the patient's weight as a dosing guideline, administer 1 gram of activated charcoal per kilogram of patient weight.

27. a. Before administering the activated charcoal, shake the container vigorously to thoroughly mix the charcoal with the water. Although it does not have a particularly bad taste, do not tell the patient it tastes good (they may not agree after trying it).

28. d. Black stools are a normal side effect of activated charcoal.

29. c. If the patient vomits shortly after taking activated charcoal, the EMT may repeat the dose one time.

30. a. Conduction refers to heat transfer through the direct contact of two objects. Convection refers to heat transfer through the movement of liquids or gases.

31. c. A patient with a spinal injury may be more at risk for hypothermia because such injury can affect the body's ability to regulate heat. Any unresponsive patient found in a cool environment should also be checked for hypothermia.

32. d. Infants and children are more at risk for hypothermia because they have small muscle mass and therefore cannot shiver as efficiently as adults. Also, they have a larger body surface area than adults and less body fat. Younger children may not be able to put on additional clothes by themselves when they get cold.

33. a. Feel the patient's abdominal skin to get a more accurate assessment of the patient's core temperature.

34. c. Depending on the core temperature of the hypothermic patient, shivering may or may not be present. Shivering ceases after the core temperature drops below 90 degrees. Shivering is usually good since it is one way the body produces heat.

35. d. In the early stages of hypothermia, the patient presents with a rapid pulse rate and rapid breathing.

36. c. Alcoholic beverages should never be given to a hypothermic patient. Alcohol produces vasodilatation that, although giving the patient a transient sense of warmth, actually increases heat loss.

37. b. Although protocols regarding treatment of hypothermic patients vary, a patient who is alert and responding appropriately can be rewarmed by applying heat packs or hot-water bottles to the groin, armpits, and neck area. These are vascular areas and warm blood is therefore pumped to all parts of the body. Use of warm oxygen also helps. Do not massage the patient, have the patient walk, or give stimulants to drink.

38. c. Hypothermic patients must be handled gently. A particular danger associated with rough handling or incorrect rewarming procedures is core temperature afterdrop. Cold, stale, highly acidic blood from the extremities may suddenly flood the core, causing cardiac arrest and death. Placement of airway adjuncts or hyperventilation may also cause cardiac arrest. However, if a pulse cannot be felt, cardiac compressions must be performed.

39. d. The pulse of a severely hypothermic patient may be hard to detect. Check the carotid pulse for 30–45 seconds before beginning CPR. Avoid the radial pulse because circulation to the extremities is impaired, making it even more difficult to detect a pulse in these areas.

40. b. Hypothermic patients are cold to the touch, may display muscle rigidity, and may appear to be dead. A hypothermic patient is not dead, however, until he or she is warm and dead. Prolonged resuscitation times, which allow for controlled rewarming in the hospital, may be necessary, but the outcome may be positive.

41. **a.** An early or superficial local cold injury may be characterized by blanching of the skin and loss of feeling and sensation in the injured area. The skin remains soft.

42. **c.** When a late or deep local cold injury occurs, the skin is white and waxy in appearance. When palpated, it will feel firm to frozen. Swelling or blisters may be present.

43. **a.** If an extremity incurs a superficial local cold injury, it should be splinted. Cover the injured area. Do not rub or massage the area or allow it to be reexposed to the cold.

44. **c.** Cover a deep cold injury with dry dressings. Do not break any blisters, rub or massage the area, apply heat to the area, or rewarm it.

45. **b.** A local cold injury may need to be rewarmed if an extremely long or delayed transport time is inevitable. However, it should not be done if the area is likely to refreeze or simply because the patient is unresponsive.

46. **d.** Rewarming should be accomplished rapidly by immersing the injured area in warm water. Continually stir the water to ensure it does not cool due to the temperature of the frozen part. Do not allow the area to refreeze. The patient will complain of severe pain.

47. **a.** When dressing hands or feet after rewarming, each finger or toe should be separated with dry, sterile dressings to prevent them from sticking together.

48. **b.** High relative humidity and high ambient temperature reduce the body's ability to dissipate heat.

49. **d.** The elderly are particularly susceptible to heat emergencies because they have poor thermoregulation and may be on many medications that affect the body's ability to dissipate heat. Although the elderly will likely be capable of removing their own clothing, they may not be able to leave a hot environment.

50. **a.** After ensuring that the patient has a adequate airway, remove the patient from the hot environment and place him or her in a cool environment.

51. **b.** Many sources link the muscle cramps that may accompany a heat emergency with a loss of body salts. Dehydration may also be a factor.

52. **d.** A dire emergency exists if a patient has dry or moist, hot temperature skin, as this indicates that the body's temperature-regulating mechanism has malfunctioned. The patient may then suffer rapid brain damage and death.

53. **c.** A responsive patient with moist, pale, normal to cool temperature skin should be encouraged to drink water. Do not give water simply because the patient is complaining of thirst. Water should not be given if the patient is nauseated or semiresponsive.

54. **d.** A patient with skin that is hot to the touch must be cooled rapidly. Cool packs can be applied to the areas of the neck, groin, and armpits to cool the patient's blood. The patient's clothing should be removed. Wetting the patient's skin with sponges or wet towels also helps dissipate body heat.

55. **c.** Near-drowning patients survive at least temporarily after the incident. They may die later, however, usually from respiratory complications.

56. **b.** Early respiratory and circulatory support are of utmost importance when managing a drowning or near-drowning patient.

57. **a.** Patients who are found unconscious in swimming pools should be suspected of having spinal injuries caused by diving into the pool.

58. **d.** A patient who is face down in a pool must be rolled face up while spinal support is provided and maintained. Ventilation should be started immediately. Chest compressions should only be performed in the water if the EMT has special training in the technique.

59. **c.** A cold water, near-drowning patient may survive a long period of immersion, far greater than 30 minutes. The EMT should attempt resuscitation. Do not try to rewarm the patient in the field. If properly managed, the patient may experience total recovery with little or no brain damage.

60. **a.** If spinal injury is not suspected, place the breathing near-drowning patient on the left side to facilitate drainage of water, vomitus, and other secretions from the upper airways.

61. **b.** If gastric distention interferes with artificial ventilation, have suction ready and place the patient on his or her left side. Apply firm pressure over the epigastric area of the abdomen to relieve distention.

62. **a.** Stingers should be scraped off using something like the edge of a card. Avoid using tweezers or forceps as these can force more venom out of the venom sac and into the patient.

63. **d.** If possible, place the injection site slightly below the level of the patient's heart to prevent the poison from reaching central circulation.

64. **b.** Generally, do not apply cold to the area of a snakebite unless ordered to do so by medical direction. Also, avoid applying heat, elevating an extremity, or allowing the patient to move around, as such actions will spread the poison.

65. **c.** When treating a snakebite, constricting bands should be used only when ordered by medical direction.

66. **c.** The EMT should always be alert for signs and symptoms of an allergic reaction and treat them accordingly.

CHAPTER 8

BEHAVIORAL EMERGENCIES

1. A behavioral emergency is when a patient:
   a. feels sad and depressed
   b. exhibits abnormal behavior that is intolerable to the patient, family, or community
   c. is disoriented and unsure of where he or she is or what day it is
   d. is under the influence of alcohol or drugs

2. Common causes for behavior alteration include:
   a. traumatic injuries
   b. low blood sugar
   c. acute illness and lack of oxygen
   d. all of the above

3. A patient experiencing a behavioral emergency in which he or she has lost touch with reality is referred to as displaying:
   a. neurotic thinking
   b. psychogenic thinking
   c. psychotic thinking
   d. neurogenic thinking

4. Patients experiencing a behavioral emergency:
   a. have psychologic and not physical problems
   b. may have an underlying physical condition causing the abnormal behavior
   c. pose little danger to the EMT if they appear calm
   d. could cope with their problems if they really wanted to

5. When dealing with a patient who is experiencing a behavioral emergency:
   a. lie to the patient if necessary
   b. tell the patient to "snap out of it"
   c. act in a calm, reassuring manner and always be honest
   d. speak in a commanding, authoritarian tone

6. When evaluating the scene of a behavioral emergency, the EMT should be particularly alert for the presence of:
   a. clutter or poor housekeeping
   b. uneaten food on the table
   c. a pet or signs of a pet
   d. unsafe objects

7. An EMT may best be able to determine if a patient's behavior is abnormal or if there is a history of violence by talking to:
   a. family members
   b. the patient himself
   c. police officers
   d. medical direction

8. Types of patients with special communication needs include:
   a. pediatric patients
   b. geriatric patients
   c. the hearing impaired
   d. all of the above

9. If a patient is displaying disturbed or abnormal thinking, such as verbalizing hallucinations:
   a. continue to treat the patient in a respectful manner
   b. go along with the situation to avoid agitating the patient
   c. explain to the patient that it is all in his or her imagination
   d. forcibly restrain the patient before transporting

10. Patients threatening suicide are at particular risk if they:
    a. are married
    b. have no history of suicidal behavior
    c. have a vague plan of action
    d. are over 40

11. When dealing with a suicidal patient, the EMT should remember that:
    a. any suicidal act or gesture should be taken seriously
    b. people who talk about suicide do not carry out the threat
    c. a patient cannot be prevented from committing suicide
    d. all of the above

12. When managing a patient who is actively threatening suicide, the course of action may include:
    a. encouraging the patient to think about alternatives and the effects the suicide may have on others
    b. daring the patient to do it to shock him or her into reality
    c. allowing the patient to remain with family members if the suicidal feelings pass
    d. telling the patient he or she doesn't really want to commit suicide

13. Conversation with a suicidal patient may include:
    a. asking why the patient thinks that suicide is the only recourse
    b. talking specifically about the patient's intentions
    c. asking the patient about any conflicts they may feel about committing suicide
    d. all of the above

14. A potential sign of violence on the part of an emotionally disturbed patient is:
    a. sitting on the edge of a seat
    b. laying on a bed or couch
    c. exhibiting open hands
    d. using monotone speech

15. To help calm an agitated patient:
    a. put your arm around the patient for reassurance
    b. maintain eye contact
    c. give the patient some time alone to regain composure
    d. avoid any slow, deliberate movements

16. Reasonable force is the amount of force it takes to:
    a. punish a patient for his or her behavior
    b. cause injury to the patient
    c. make the patient do as the EMT says
    d. prevent the patient from injuring himself or herself or others

17. The amount of reasonable force that an EMT uses depends on the:
    a. patient's vital signs
    b. patient's size
    c. amount of vulgarity the patient uses
    d. type of clothing the patient is wearing

18. If a violent patient is encountered, the best course of action is to:
    a. approach the patient alone to gain his or her confidence
    b. surprise the patient and overpower him or her
    c. approach the patient only with backup assistance
    d. threaten the patient with bodily harm if he or she does not cooperate

19. Restraints should be used on patients:
    a. who pose a danger to themselves or others
    b. with a history of serious behavioral problems
    c. who have committed a crime
    d. who are injured and intoxicated but refuse to go to the hospital

20. Generally, the minimum number of persons needed to restrain a patient is:
   a. two
   b. three
   c. four
   d. five

21. When approaching a patient who is about to be restrained:
   a. do not speak to the patient during the restraining process
   b. only one rescuer at a time should approach the patient
   c. all the rescuers should approach at the same time
   d. one EMT should carry a weapon to use in case the patient overpowers the other rescuers

22. The recommended position in which a restrained patient should be placed is:
   a. on the right side
   b. on the left side
   c. face down
   d. the Trendelenburg position

23. After restraints are applied, the EMT should:
   a. remove them if the patient agrees not to cause further trouble
   b. not remove or loosen them before reaching the hospital
   c. remove only the wrist restraints if the patient agrees not to cause further trouble
   d. not remove the restraints but frequently reassess circulation

24. If the patient starts spitting on the EMTs:
   a. cover the patient's face with a surgical mask
   b. use surgical tape to tape the patient's mouth closed
   c. place a pillow over the patient's face
   d. use a cravat to tie the patient's jaw shut

25. When transporting a female patient who is experiencing a behavioral emergency:
   a. a male EMT should ride with the patient
   b. the patient should never be restrained
   c. a female EMT should ride with the patient if possible
   d. a police officer should accompany the EMTs

26. When documenting a situation in which restraints were used:
   a. avoid implying that the patient was violent, as this could be considered slander
   b. note the techniques used to restrain the patient
   c. record word for word any abusive speech directed toward the EMTs
   d. all of the above

ADDITIONAL POINTS FOR DISCUSSION

1. What is your local Suicide Prevention phone number?

2. To which hospital(s) would you normally transport a behavioral emergency patient?

3. What are your department's policies regarding transportation of violent patients?

4. What types of restraints are carried on your ambulance? Review the procedure for using each piece.

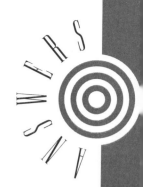
8 BEHAVIORAL EMERGENCIES

1. **b.** A behavioral emergency is when a patient exhibits abnormal behavior that is intolerable to the patient, family, or community. Some people, such as elderly persons, may be disoriented to place and time but may not be experiencing a behavioral emergency.

2. **d.** All of the above. There are a number of common causes for behavioral emergencies, including psychogenic problems or the use of mind-altering substances. Medical causes can include traumatic injuries, low blood sugar, lack of oxygen, and illness.

3. **c.** Psychotic thinking is marked by loss of touch with reality and is frequently accompanied by delusions or hallucinations.

4. **b.** EMTs must remember that behavioral emergencies may be caused by physical conditions, such as low oxygen or low blood sugar, as well as by psychologic reasons. In either case, the EMT should use caution because of the potential for danger.

5. **c.** Act in a calm, reassuring manner when dealing with behavioral emergencies. Never lie to the patient or speak in an authoritarian manner.

6. **d.** EMTs should be particularly alert for the presence of unsafe objects that could be used as weapons. Such objects may either be in the patient's possession or within the patient's reach.

7. **a.** The family and sometimes bystanders who are familiar with the patient's history are the best resource for an EMT to determine if a patient's behavior is abnormal. These individuals may also be able to provide information on the patient's potential for violence. The patient may usually display what the EMT would consider to be abnormal behavior—the question is, what is different about the behavior at this time that warrants intervention by EMTs? Although police officers may not be familiar with the patient, they may provide helpful information if they have dealt with the patient before.

8. **d.** All of the above. Types of patients with special communication needs include pediatric, geriatric, and disabled patients, including those with hearing or visual impairment. Non-English speaking patients may also have special communication needs. Communication problems may be mistaken for behavioral problems by the EMT.

9. **a.** A patient should always be treated in a respectful manner, even if they are displaying signs of disturbed or abnormal thinking. Do not go along with the situation or try to argue with the patient. Restraint is usually unnecessary unless the patient is a danger to himself or herself or others.

10. d. Patients who are over 40 are at a higher risk for suicide. Other risk factors include being widowed, single, divorced, or having a history of depression or alcoholism. A defined plan of action, easy access to lethal means, and a previous history of self-destructive behavior also place the patient in a high-risk category for suicide.

11. a. Any suicidal act or gesture must be taken seriously. People who talk about suicide do commit suicide. With proper care, the patient may be helped through a suicidal crisis.

12. a. A patient may be encouraged to think about alternatives to suicide. Getting the patient to think about how the suicide will affect others who care may also help. Do not dare the patient to commit suicide. Some patients sincerely want to commit suicide, and telling them that they don't may make them believe that their feelings are not important.

13. d. All of the above. Ask the patient why he or she feels that suicide is the only recourse. Don't be afraid to talk specifically about the patient's intentions of committing suicide or how they feel about it.

14. a. The patient's posture and actions can do much to alert an EMT to potential violence. The patient may be sitting on the edge of a seat, swearing and yelling, or clenching the fists. Any behavior displayed by the patient that makes the EMT feel uneasy should be taken seriously.

15. b. It is important to maintain eye contact when trying to calm a patient. Remain a comfortable distance from the patient when talking, and avoid sudden movements. Do not leave the patient alone.

16. d. Reasonable force is the amount of force it takes to prevent a patient from injuring himself or herself or others. Force should not be used as a means of telling the patient that the EMT is in control or be used as a form of punishment. Force should be used in a manner that does not injure the patient.

17. b. The amount of reasonable force that an EMT uses depends on the patient's size. Other factors to be taken into account include sex, mental state, the type of abnormal behavior being displayed, and the method of restraint to be used. Behavioral emergency patients are often uncooperative and will not allow EMTs to obtain vital signs.

18. c. Never approach a violent patient alone. Have backup assistance, preferably that of the police. If a patient has a weapon, let the police handle the situation. Do not surprise or threaten the patient.

19. a. The policy for use of restraints varies from area to area. Generally, they should be used if the patient poses a physical threat to himself or herself or others. Once the patient has been restrained, do not let him or her out of the restraints until the patient reaches the hospital.

20. c. Generally, at least four people, one assigned to each limb, are needed to restrain a patient. More people can be used if available. Law-enforcement personnel and medical direction should be consulted prior to restraining the patient.

21. c. Everyone involved in restraining the patient should approach at the same time. One EMT should talk to the patient during the restraining process. EMTs should not use weapons on the patient.

22. **c.** After securing the patient's limbs, it is generally recommended that the patient be positioned face down on the stretcher unless injuries dictate otherwise. Some areas recommend positioning the patient face up. Always follow your local protocols.

23. **d.** Restraints on the wrists and ankles can impair circulation, so frequently reassess circulation in the hands and feet. Loosen restraints if circulation is impaired, but do not remove them. Once restraints have been applied they should not be released until after the patient reaches the receiving facility.

24. **a.** If the patient is spitting on the rescuers, place a surgical mask over the patient's face. Do not do anything that could interfere with the airway or create a problem in the event that the patient vomits.

25. **c.** It is desirable to have a female EMT ride with a female patient who is experiencing a behavioral emergency. If the patient is violent, restraints may be necessary. Although police may be involved, local protocol will dictate whether a law enforcement officer must accompany the EMTs and the patient.

26. **b.** Documentation is critical when a patient has been restrained. Note the reason restraints were necessary, the type of restraints used, and the technique used to restrain the patient. If the patient was violent, this should be clearly noted as it is part of the reason the patient was restrained. It is not necessary to document the patient's speech word for word. Recording the use of abusive language toward the EMTs is sufficient.

OBSTETRICS AND GYNECOLOGY

1. The structure in which a fetus grows and develops is the:
   a. fallopian tube
   b. vagina
   c. uterus
   d. ovary

2. The bag of water that protects the baby is called the:
   a. afterbirth
   b. alkalotic pack
   c. uterine envelope
   d. amniotic sac

3. The placenta:
   a. mixes the baby's blood with the mother's
   b. exchanges oxygen, nutrients, and waste products between the mother and fetus
   c. is used by the fetus for food
   d. is normally positioned in the uterus over the cervix

4. The cervix is the:
   a. wall of the endothelium
   b. neck of the uterus
   c. lower portion of the endometrium
   d. distal end of the perineum

5. The area of skin between the vagina and the anus that can tear during delivery is the:
   a. perineum
   b. periosteum
   c. peritoneum
   d. pericardium

6. When a pregnant patient is encountered, questions would include:
   a. when the baby is due
   b. whether the patient is experiencing any pains or contractions
   c. whether there is any bleeding or discharge, and when it began
   d. all of the above

7. Questions concerning the patient's pains would normally include all of the following *except*:
   a. when the pain began
   b. how far apart the pains are
   c. whether the pain is aggravated by movement
   d. the duration of the pain

8. The first stage of labor covers the period from:
   a. when the ambulance is called until the arrival of the EMTs
   b. when regular contractions begin to when the baby enters the birth canal
   c. the patient's first contractions to the delivery of the baby's head
   d. dilatation of the cervix to the birth of the baby

9. The EMT should consider delivery imminent when:
   a. contractions are less than 2 minutes apart
   b. contractions last longer than 20 seconds
   c. it is the mother's first pregnancy and contractions are 5 minutes apart
   d. the patient is experiencing lower abdominal pain with no back pain

10. When the head of the baby bulges against the vaginal opening, this is known as:
    a. presenting
    b. crowning
    c. birthing
    d. showing

11. The second stage of labor covers the period from:
    a. delivery of the baby's head to delivery of the placenta
    b. arrival of the ambulance to the start of transport
    c. when the baby enters the birth canal to the birth of the baby
    d. the end of contractions to the presentation of the baby's head

12. The third stage of labor covers the period:
    a. from dilatation of the cervix to delivery of the placenta
    b. from the arrival at the hospital to transfer to the obstetrics ward
    c. following the birth of the baby through delivery of the placenta
    d. following delivery of the baby to arrival at the hospital

13. An EMT should insert his or her fingers into a pregnant patient's vagina:
    a. to support the baby's head during delivery
    b. only in the case of a breech delivery or prolapsed cord
    c. to assist in delivery of the baby's shoulders
    d. to check the baby's pulse in the case of a limb presentation

14. Immediately following delivery of the baby's head, all of the following should be done *except:*
    a. stimulating breathing
    b. checking if the umbilical cord is around the baby's neck
    c. checking to be sure the amniotic sac is not covering the baby's mouth and nostrils
    d. suctioning the mouth and nostrils

15. When suctioning a newborn:
    a. wait until delivery is complete to begin
    b. squeeze the bulb syringe after inserting it
    c. insert the tip of the bulb syringe 2–3 inches into the mouth and each nostril
    d. squeeze the bulb syringe before inserting it

16. The first place the EMT should suction the newborn is:
    a. the right nostril
    b. the left nostril
    c. the mouth
    d. either the mouth or nostrils

17. A major concern when caring for a newborn is:
    a. starting the mother-infant bonding process
    b. wrapping the newborn in moist towels
    c. guarding against heat loss
    d. breathing rates greater than 30 breaths per minute

18. To stimulate the baby to breathe:
    a. hold it upside-down by its feet and ankles
    b. gently rub its back or flick the soles of its feet
    c. slap it sharply on the buttocks
    d. use an oxygen-powered resuscitator

Sign	0	1	2
Appearance (Skin color)	bluish or pale	pink or typical newborn color; hands and feet are blue	pink or typical newborn color; entire body
Pulse (Heart rate)	absent	below 100	over 100
Grimace (Irritability)	no response	crying; some motion	crying; vigorous
Activity (Muscle tone)	limp	some flexion—extremities	active; good motion in extremities
Respiratory effort	absent	slow and irregular	normal; crying

Figure 9-1   APGAR Scale.

19. After delivery is completed but before the cord is cut, the baby should be positioned:
   a. at the same level as the mother's vagina
   b. higher than the mother
   c. with the head slightly elevated
   d. lower than the mother

20. The proper time to cut the umbilical cord is:
   a. after delivery of the placenta
   b. 10–15 minutes after delivery
   c. before the infant starts to breathe
   d. after pulsations in the cord cease

21. If a decision is made to cut the umbilical cord, the first clamp should be placed about:
   a. 5 inches from the baby
   b. 5 inches from the mother
   c. 10 inches from the baby
   d. 10 inches from the mother

22. After the cord is cut, the baby should be positioned:
   a. on the right side
   b. with the head slightly higher than the trunk
   c. in a prone position
   d. with the head slightly lower than the trunk

 23. An assessment of APGAR should be made:
   a. immediately following delivery and upon reaching the hospital
   b. 1 and 5 minutes after birth
   c. 5 and 10 minutes after birth
   d. immediately following delivery and 10 minutes later

For questions 24 and 25, refer to the APGAR scale in Figure 9-1

 24. A newborn presents with some pink skin color, a pulse rate of 140, a weak cry, good muscle tone, and breathing rate of 36. The APGAR score is:
   a. 6
   b. 7
   c. 8
   d. 9

25. A baby was delivered by its father 3 minutes prior to the EMS unit's arrival. He is cyanotic, has a pulse rate of 106, a weak cry, no muscle tone, and breathing rate of 18. The APGAR score is:
   a. 3
   b. 4
   c. 5
   d. 6

26. If the newborn is breathing but his or her heart rate is below 100:
    a. start artificial ventilation
    b. flick the soles of the feet
    c. start chest compressions only
    d. perform CPR

27. The placenta should deliver:
    a. 30–45 minutes after birth
    b. immediately after the cord is cut
    c. 1 hour after birth
    d. within 20 minutes of birth

28. After the placenta has been delivered:
    a. wrap it in a towel, place it in a plastic bag, and take it to the hospital with the mother
    b. discard it
    c. have the mother walk to induce uterine contractions
    d. sit the mother in an upright position

29. During childbirth, a patient may normally experience blood loss up to:
    a. 500 cc
    b. 5 cups
    c. 2 pints
    d. 1 liter

30. Excessive maternal bleeding after delivery may be managed in all of the following ways *except:*
    a. massaging the mother's lower abdomen
    b. packing the vagina with a sterile dressing
    c. having the baby suckle
    d. placing a sterile pad over the vaginal opening

31. A newborn is considered premature if he or she:
    a. is born before the ninth month of pregnancy
    b. weighs more than 6 pounds
    c. delivers before 28 weeks (7 months) of gestation
    d. weighs less than 7½ pounds

32. Regarding premature infants:
    a. do not give oxygen because it will cause blindness
    b. the head is small in proportion to the rest of the body
    c. do not suction the mouth or nose because it can cause excessive drying of the mucous membranes
    d. they are at risk for hypothermia

33. Breech presentation refers to an abnormal delivery in which:
    a. the baby's shoulders are too large to pass through the birth canal
    b. the amniotic sac fails to rupture
    c. the baby's buttocks deliver first
    d. the umbilical cord is wrapped around the baby's neck

34. Management of a breech delivery may include:
    a. pulling on the baby
    b. placing two gloved fingers in the vagina to form an airway for the baby
    c. having the mother cross her legs to delay delivery
    d. placing the hand over the vaginal orifice to prevent delivery

35. In a situation involving a prolapsed cord, breech presentation, or limb presentation, the mother may be placed:
    a. in a head-down position with the pelvis elevated
    b. on the right side with the legs squeezed together
    c. in a prone position
    d. on the back with the head higher than the feet

36. When examining the mother, if a prolapse cord is discovered:
    a. do not allow anything to touch the cord
    b. attempt to push the cord back into the vagina and uterus
    c. insert several gloved fingers into the vagina and gently push on the baby's head to relieve pressure on the cord
    d. pull on the cord to induce delivery

37. Delivery involving a limb presentation would include:
   a. attempting to push the limb back into the uterus
   b. encouraging the mother to push
   c. pulling on the limb to assist delivery
   d. immediately transporting to the hospital

38. The presence of meconium indicates:
   a. a lack of lubricating fluid in the birth canal
   b. possible fetal distress during labor
   c. an abnormal passage of the baby through the birth canal
   d. the probability of a breech presentation

39. The primary problems associated with a meconium emergency are:
   a. cardiac complications
   b. neurologic complications
   c. breathing complications
   d. intestinal complications

✱ 40. The most common cause of fetal death is:
   a. maternal death
   b. drug abuse by the mother
   c. strangulation by the umbilical cord
   d. suffocation by the amniotic sac

✱ 41. When caring for an injured, pregnant patient, the general rule is:
   a. do not waste time packaging the patient if delivery is imminent
   b. that the life of the unborn child takes precedence over the life of the mother
   c. that the life of the mother takes precedence over the life of the unborn child
   d. that there is little concern unless the patient is near term

42. When a pregnant patient with a spinal injury is transported on a backboard, the backboard should:
   a. be tilted to the right
   b. be tilted to the left
   c. have the head elevated
   d. be completely flat

43. Vaginal bleeding occurring during late pregnancy usually indicates:
   a. imminent birth
   b. a problem with the placenta
   c. the possibility that seizures will occur
   d. a probable multiple-birth situation

44. Abnormally low blood pressure in a pregnant patient may be caused by:
   a. toxemia of pregnancy
   b. compression of the aorta by the baby
   c. premature uterine contractions
   d. compression of the vena cava by the baby

45. The EMT should be alert for the possibility of seizures when a pregnant patient presents with:
   a. swelling of the face, hands, and feet
   b. abnormally low blood pressure
   c. sudden loss of weight
   d. severe lower abdominal pain

✱ 46. After seizures are experienced by a pregnant patient, the patient should be transported:
   a. in a supine position
   b. rapidly with red light and siren
   c. with the legs and feet elevated
   d. with the shoulders and head elevated

47. Miscarriage refers to:
   a. delivery of the fetus before it can live independently of the mother
   b. self-induced termination of pregnancy
   c. bleeding that occurs before the 37th week of pregnancy
   d. misplacement of the placenta on the uterine wall

48. An important part of managing a miscarriage includes:
   a. discarding fetal tissues to avoid disturbing the mother
   b. advising the patient to make an appointment with her obstetrician
   c. rendering emotional support to the mother and father
   d. transporting the patient positioned on the left side with the head elevated as if she were in shock

49. The soft areas in a baby's head where the fusion of the bones of the skull is not complete are known as:
    a. fontanelles
    b. varices
    c. foramens
    d. parietes

50. When approaching a sexual assault patient:
    a. tell the patient how the assault could have been avoided
    b. reassure the patient
    c. tell the patient everything will be all right
    d. avoid any physical examination

51. To appropriately care for a sexual assault patient:
    a. be careful to preserve any evidence
    b. allow the patient to wash and change clothes
    c. get as much information as possible about the incident
    d. allow the patient to go to the bathroom

52. If it is necessary to transport a female patient injured in a sexual assault:
    a. a male EMT should ride with the patient
    b. the patient should be restrained
    c. a female EMT should ride with the patient if possible
    d. it is better to send the patient to the hospital in a police car

53. Documentation of a sexual assault on an EMS report should include:
    a. the EMTs' personal opinions about the incident
    b. what the patient has said as well as what is observed
    c. theories regarding who the EMT thinks may be involved
    d. all of the above

ADDITIONAL POINTS FOR DISCUSSION

1. Review the equipment carried in your OB kits and each piece's use.

2. Is there a specific hospital in your area that is used to treat and examine victims of sexual assault? If so, which?

3. Review any special procedures involving patient management and crime scene preservation that should be followed at the scene of a sexual assault with your local law enforcement agency.

4. What is your local Rape Crisis Hotline phone number?

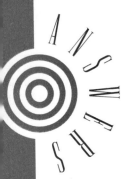

9 OBSTETRICS AND GYNECOLOGY

1. **c.** The uterus is a muscular organ in which the fetus grows and develops. The ovaries produce sex hormones and ova. Ova are carried from the ovaries to the uterus by the fallopian tubes. The vagina is the lower part of the birth canal.

2. **d.** The amniotic sac protects the infant in the uterus. Afterbirth is another term for the placenta.

3. **b.** The placenta exchanges oxygen, nutrients, and waste products between the mother and the fetus. It is normally positioned high in the uterus and does not allow mixing of the baby's blood with the mother's.

4. **b.** The cervix is the neck of the uterus.

5. **a.** The perineum is the area of skin between the vagina and the anus. During delivery, the skin in this area may tear due to the pressure exerted by the fetus as it passes through the birth canal. The periosteum is a fiberlike covering of the bones, the pericardium is the sac around the heart, and the peritoneum is the membrane lining the abdominal cavity.

6. **d.** All of the above. An obstetrics patient should be questioned concerning when the baby is due and if the patient is experiencing any pains or contractions. Ask if she has been experiencing any bleeding or discharge, such as if the water has broken, and if so, when.

7. **c.** Question the patient concerning how far apart her labor pains are and the duration of the pain. It is also helpful to know when the pain started.

8. **b.** The first stage of labor covers the period from the beginning of regular contractions to when the baby enters the birth canal.

9. **a.** Consider delivery imminent if contractions are less than 2 minutes apart or if the baby is crowning. Labor during a first delivery is longer than subsequent deliveries. Transport unless delivery is expected within 5 minutes. Remember, there are worse places to deliver a baby than in the back of an ambulance, so don't be afraid to transport.

10. **b.** Crowning is the term used for when the baby's head bulges against the vaginal opening.

11. **c.** The second stage of labor covers the period from when the baby enters the birth canal to the birth of the baby.

12. **c.** The third stage of labor covers the period following the birth of the baby through delivery of the placenta.

13. b. There are only two cases in which an EMT should insert fingers into a pregnant patient's vagina: 1) in the case of a breech birth to form an airway, and 2) in the case of a prolapsed cord to relieve pressure on the cord. Always wear sterile gloves to diminish the risk of transmitting infection.

14. a. Immediately following delivery of the baby's head is not the time to stimulate breathing. It is the time to check for the umbilical cord around the baby's neck, check to ensure that the amniotic sac is not in place over the baby's head and face, and to suction the mouth and nose. If the amniotic sac is not broken, puncture it and push it away from the newborn's head and mouth.

15. d. Always squeeze the bulb syringe before inserting, and insert it only 1–1½ inches into the mouth and nostrils. Suction should be applied immediately.

16. c. The EMT should first suction the mouth of the newborn and then the nostrils. This prevents aspiration of matter in the mouth in the event that spontaneous breathing is stimulated by suctioning the nostrils.

17. c. The EMT must guard against heat loss in a newborn. Quickly dry the infant, and wrap it in a warm blanket. Since the head is so large, a covering (such as a stockinette) should always be placed over the head to diminish heat loss. Breathing rates greater than 30 breaths a minute are normal in the newborn.

18. b. Breathing may be stimulated by gently rubbing the baby's back or tapping the soles of its feet. Do not hold it upside-down, slap it, or use an oxygen-powered breathing device.

19. a. Following delivery, the baby should be kept level with the mother's vagina until the cord is clamped and cut. Positioning the baby too high may cause hypovolemia, as blood is siphoned back into the placenta. Placing the baby too low may cause fluid overload.

20. d. After pulsations in the umbilical cord cease, it should be clamped and cut.

21. c. The first umbilical clamp should be placed about 10 inches away from the baby. The second clamp is then placed about 3 inches closer to the baby. Cut between the clamps.

22. d. After the cord is cut, position the baby with its head slightly lower than its trunk to facilitate drainage of fluids from its mouth and nose.

23. b. An assessment of APGAR should be made 1 minute and 5 minutes after birth. APGAR is an acronym for: *A*ppearance, *P*ulse, *G*rimace, *A*ctivity, and *R*espiratory effort.

24. c. The patient's score is 8: Appearance = 1, Pulse = 2, Grimace = 1, Activity = 2, Respiratory effort = 2).

25. b. The patient's score is 4: Appearance = 0, Pulse = 2, Grimace = 1, Activity = 0, Respiratory effort = 1).

26. a. Start artificial ventilation if the newborn's heart rate drops below 100 beats per minute. Low heart rates are often a result of low oxygenation, so good ventilation can actually increase the infant's heart rate. If the heart rate drops below 80 beats per minute, start chest compressions also.

27. **d.** The placenta should normally deliver in about 20 minutes, but may take up to 30 minutes.

28. **a.** The placenta should be wrapped in a towel, then placed in a plastic bag, and taken to the hospital for examination. Do not have the patient squeeze her legs together or walk around.

29. **a.** Blood loss of 500 cc may be normal during childbirth.

30. **b.** Maternal bleeding may be managed by massaging the patient's abdomen, having the baby suckle, or placing the patient in the shock position with a sterile pad over the vaginal opening. Never pack the vagina.

31. **c.** A baby born before 28 weeks (7 months) of gestation or one that weighs less than 5½ pounds is considered premature. Normal newborns weigh about 7 pounds.

32. **d.** Premature babies are very susceptible to hypothermia. If oxygen is given over a short period it should not cause complications, but the stream should not be directed at the baby's face. The head is usually larger, and suctioning may need to be repeated frequently because the airways can easily become obstructed.

33. **c.** A breech presentation occurs when the baby's buttocks or lower extremities are low in the uterus and deliver first.

34. **b.** It may be necessary to place two gloved fingers in the mother's vagina to form an airway for the baby. Do not pull on the baby or in any way attempt to delay delivery.

35. **a.** Patients may be placed in a head-down position with the hips elevated when such obstetric emergencies as breech or limb presentation or a prolapsed cord are encountered.

36. **c.** Management of a prolapsed umbilical cord may include inserting several gloved fingers into the vagina and gently pushing on the baby's head to relieve the pressure on the cord. Do not attempt to push the cord back into the vagina. Any exposed portion of cord should be covered with moist, sterile dressings.

37. **d.** In the case of a limb presentation, immediate transportation to the hospital is of utmost importance.

38. **b.** The presence of meconium (the dark-green contents of the intestines of a newborn child) indicates possible fetal distress during labor. If the infant has a bowel movement and passes the meconium before birth, it mixes with the amniotic fluid and forms a liquid that resembles thick, dark green pea soup.

39. **c.** The presence of meconium in amniotic fluid denotes a true emergency. If the infant aspirates meconium, breathing complications may be serious to fatal. If a meconium emergency exists, rapid transportation to a hospital is warranted. Take extra care to fully suction the infant.

40. **a.** Maternal death is the most common cause of fetal death. If the mother dies from trauma, perform CPR and transport her to a hospital. A physician may be able to perform an emergency caesarean section to save the infant.

41. **c.** The general rule is that the life of the mother takes precedence over the life of the unborn child.

42. b. When transporting an injured pregnant female on a backboard, the backboard should be tilted to the left. This relieves the pressure that the fetus may place on the vena cava, which is the major blood vessel in the abdomen.

43. b. Vaginal bleeding occurring during late pregnancy usually indicates a problem with the placenta. The bleeding may or may not be accompanied by pain.

44. d. Compression of the mother's vena cava (the vein that returns blood from the lower body to the heart) by the baby in the uterus can cause abnormally low blood pressure. If this is suspected, transport the patient on her left side to take pressure off the vessel.

45. a. Swelling of the face, hands, and feet of a pregnant patient should alert the EMT to the possibility of seizures. Also, the patient may have an elevated blood pressure and a recent history of sudden weight gain.

46. d. After a pregnant patient has experienced seizures, she should be transported with the shoulders and head elevated. Use of the ambulance siren should be avoided as it may precipitate additional seizures.

47. a. Miscarriage refers to the delivery of the fetus before it can live independently of the mother.

48. c. An important part of managing a miscarriage includes providing emotional support to the parents. Tissues should be taken to the hospital for examination. Because the EMT cannot adequately assess the patient's uterus, the patient should be evaluated at a hospital. If the patient displays signs of hypoperfusion, transport her on her back with her legs elevated.

49. a. The fontanelles are soft areas in a baby's head where the cranial bones have not fused together. The EMT must exercise care to prevent pushing on these areas while managing the infant's head during normal or abnormal delivery.

50. b. Always act in a professional, reassuring manner. Do not tell the patient how the assault could have been avoided or that everything will be all right. The patient should be examined, but the exam may have to be altered according to the situation.

51. a. Be careful to preserve evidence at the scene and on the patient. Although the EMT cannot prohibit it, the patient should be discouraged from changing clothes, washing, or using the bathroom. EMTs are usually not police officers and should not question the patient about specifics relating to the assault.

52. c. It is desirable to have a female EMT ride with a female patient who has been sexually assaulted. Unless the patient is violent, restraints are not appropriate. Also, because the patient is injured (emotionally as well as physically), transport in a police car is not warranted.

53. b. An EMT should note only facts on the EMS report. This could include what the patient has said as well as what can be observed. This document will probably be used in court, so avoid including personal opinions or theories.

BLEEDING AND SHOCK

1. Shock may be defined as:
   a. lack of blood in the circulatory system
   b. inadequate perfusion of the body's cells and tissues
   c. inability of the heart to pump efficiently
   d. a severe allergic reaction causing internal blood loss

2. Hypoperfusion caused by bleeding is known as:
   a. hemorrhagic shock
   b. anaphylactic shock
   c. cardiogenic shock
   d. circulatory shock

3. Concerning the blood pressure of a patient in shock, remember that:
   a. a drop in blood pressure is an early sign of shock
   b. blood pressure is directly proportional to the pulse
   c. blood pressure drops initially and then rises
   d. a drop in blood pressure is a late sign of shock

4. Capillary refill time should be checked on:
   a. all hypoperfusion patients
   b. patients injured in automobile accidents
   c. trauma patients only
   d. infants and children only

5. Normal capillary refill time is:
   a. less than 2 seconds
   b. more than 3 seconds
   c. between 2 and 4 seconds
   d. less than 4 seconds

6. An early indication of shock may be:
   a. constricted pupils
   b. decreased pulse rate
   c. restlessness and anxiety
   d. dry skin

7. The key elements of the circulatory system that are needed to maintain tissue perfusion include all of the following *except*:
   a. a functioning pump (the heart)
   b. a one-way directional system (the valves in veins)
   c. adequate fluid in the system (the blood)
   d. intact pipes (the blood vessels)

8. When caring for a patient in shock:
   a. place the patient on oxygen after splinting fractures
   b. control bleeding after ensuring an adequate airway and breathing
   c. apply heating pads or hot water bottles to warm the patient
   d. check vital signs every 15 minutes

9. To place a patient in the shock position:
   a. elevate the entire body with the head higher than the feet
   b. place the patient in Trendelenburg position if no spinal injury is suspected
   c. elevate the lower extremities if no spinal injury is suspected
   d. elevate only the upper torso and head

10. Ideally, the vital signs of a patient in shock should be checked:
    a. every 5 minutes
    b. every 10 minutes
    c. every 15 minutes
    d. every 20 minutes

11. When managing a patient with severe external bleeding:
    a. control the bleeding prior to donning gloves
    b. only gloves and eye protection are needed
    c. determine whether the patient has a communicable disease prior to donning protective gear
    d. use gloves, eye protection, gown, and mask when possible

12. A serious amount of sudden blood loss in adults is:
    a. 1 unit
    b. 500 cc
    c. 1 liter
    d. 2 cups

13. Venous bleeding is:
    a. a slow flow of bright-red blood
    b. a steady ooze of blood from a wound
    c. a steady flow of dark-red blood
    d. difficult to control with direct pressure

14. Bleeding from an artery:
    a. is bright-red and spurts with each heartbeat
    b. is not life-threatening
    c. can be easily controlled by direct pressure
    d. can only be controlled with a tourniquet

15. Capillary bleeding is:
    a. associated with long clotting times
    b. slow, oozing, and dark red
    c. bright red and steady
    d. controlled by use of pressure points

16. After protective gear is donned, the first step to control bleeding is:
    a. applying direct pressure
    b. placing the patient in shock position
    c. placing digital pressure on an artery
    d. applying a cold pack

17. To provide pressure to control bleeding, all of the following may be used *except:*
    a. the PASG
    b. the hand
    c. an air splint
    d. a narrow bandage

18. Along with using direct pressure to control bleeding in an extremity:
    a. immerse the extremity in cold water
    b. lower the extremity
    c. apply ice to the wound area
    d. elevate the extremity

19. The pressure point of choice for controlling bleeding from a forearm injury is the:
    a. temporal artery
    b. popliteal artery
    c. brachial artery
    d. tibial artery

20. To manage uncontrolled bleeding from a leg injury, the pressure point of choice is the:
    a. subclavian artery
    b. radial artery
    c. plexal artery
    d. femoral artery

✱ 21. When using digital pressure on an arterial pressure point:
    a. continue to apply direct pressure to the wound
    b. alternate with 2 minutes of pressure on, 2 minutes off
    c. do not apply any pressure to the wound
    d. the artery chosen should be distal to the wound

22. A tourniquet should be used:
a. on crush injuries involving an extremity
b. only as a last resort
c. when direct pressure alone does not control bleeding
d. when an amputation is encountered

23. When a bandage is used as a tourniquet, it should be:
a. wrapped twice around the extremity
b. loosened every 20 minutes to resupply the area below with blood
c. between 1 and 2 inches wide
d. applied as far from the wound as possible

24. Tighten a tourniquet:
a. just enough to occlude venous blood flow
b. enough to occlude arterial blood flow
c. as much as possible
d. until pain below the wound is relieved

25. After applying a tourniquet:
a. document its use and the time it was applied on the EMS report
b. cover the wound and tourniquet with sterile dressings and bandages
c. lower the extremity below the level of the heart
d. apply digital pressure to the appropriate pressure point

26. A problem with using a blood-pressure cuff as a tourniquet is that:
a. it is not wide enough
b. it cannot occlude arterial blood flow
c. there is a greater likelihood of damaging underlying structures
d. it may gradually lose pressure

27. Another term for nosebleed is:
a. epinephrine
b. epiphyseal
c. epistaxis
d. epidural

28. To manage a nosebleed with no associated spinal injury:
a. apply direct pressure to the facial artery
b. have the patient lean forward
c. pack the nostril with gauze
d. have the patient lie on his or her back

29. When managing a patient with a head injury accompanied by a nosebleed:
a. pack the nose with gauze
b. pinch the nostrils, and tip the head back
c. do not attempt to stop bleeding
d. place the patient in a sitting position

✱ 30. Match the following bone injury with its associated blood loss:
femur, humerus, pelvis, rib, tibia
_____ 125 cc (¼ unit)
_____ 250 cc (½ unit)
_____ 500–750 cc (1–1½ units)
_____ 1,000 cc (2 units)
_____ 1,000–10,000 cc (2–20 units)

31. Vomiting of coffee-ground emesis may indicate:
a. appendicitis
b. bleeding from the colon
c. diverticulitis
d. internal bleeding of the stomach

32. Stools that resemble tar indicate:
a. an abdominal aneurysm
b. appendicitis
c. bleeding in the upper intestines
d. gastritis

33. Signs of internal bleeding may include all of the following *except:*
a. bright-red blood in the stool or vomitus
b. lack of thirst
c. an enlarged, tender, rigid abdomen
d. rapid, weak pulse

34. If internal bleeding is suspected, be alert for the possibility of:
a. a severe allergic reaction
b. an increase in blood pressure
c. nausea and vomiting
d. fever

35. Bilateral femur fractures may be accompanied by:
a. brachial nerve damage
b. shock, but only if associated with other internal injuries
c. moderate to severe shock
d. spasms of the Achilles tendon

36. If signs of shock are present, use of the PASG is indicated in the event of:
a. pelvic injury with signs of abdominal bleeding
b. an open wound to the chest with severe external bleeding
c. blunt trauma to the chest with signs of internal bleeding
d. isolated open head injury accompanied by severe external bleeding

37. The PASG should *not* be applied if the patient exhibits:
a. a diminished level of consciousness
b. a rapid pulse
c. signs of fluid in the lungs
d. dropping blood pressure

 38. When properly placed, the top of the PASG should lie:
a. immediately below the level of the diaphragm
b. at the nipple line
c. at the level of the umbilicus
d. at the level of the sixth rib

39. The PASG should be inflated:
a. whenever the patient's blood pressure drops below 100 systolic
b. only after approval is given by medical direction
c. whenever the patient's pulse rate exceeds 100 beats per minute
d. any of the above

40. When applying the PASG, inflate it until the:
a. patient states that he or she feels better
b. patient's blood pressure reaches 120 systolic
c. Velcro™ starts to crackle
d. pressure gauges reach 90 mm Hg

41. Deflation of the PASG should be accomplished:
a. in the field after IVs are started
b. by first deflating the legs and then the abdomen
c. slowly, stopping deflation after each blood pressure drop of 10–15 mm Hg in order to stabilize the patient with fluids
d. only by trained personnel in a clinical setting

ADDITIONAL POINTS FOR DISCUSSION

1. What are some of the ways to place the PASG on a patient?

2. What are your local protocols for use, inflation, and deflation of the PASG?

3. What procedure does your department employ for cleaning and disinfecting the PASG after use?

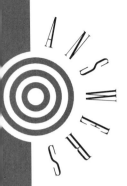

10 BLEEDING AND SHOCK

1. b. Shock is defined as inadequate perfusion of the body's cells and tissues with oxygen and nutrients as well as inadequate removal of metabolic waste products.

2. a. Hemorrhagic shock is hypoperfusion caused by blood loss.

3. d. A drop in blood pressure is a late sign of shock. Infants and children often maintain a good pressure until they are very close to death. An increase in pulse is a better indicator of shock in the early stages. The EMT must be alert to recognize shock long before blood pressure drops.

4. d. Capillary refill time should only be checked on infants and children younger than 6 years.

5. a. Normal capillary refill time in infants and children is less than 2 seconds.

6. c. Restlessness and anxiety, or a change in mental status caused by a decreased delivery of oxygen to brain tissues, may be the first indication of shock. Shock patients also develop an increased pulse rate, moist skin, and dilated pupils.

7. b. For perfusion to be maintained, there must be an intact pump (the heart), adequate fluid in the system (the blood), and intact pipes (the blood vessels). A one-way directional system is not a key element.

8. b. Airway and breathing are the first priority in managing shock. Major bleeding should be controlled, and the patient should be placed on oxygen as quickly as possible. Place the patient in the shock position and keep the patient warm, but do not overheat the patient.

9. c. The shock position involves elevating only the patient's lower extremities 8–12 inches if no spinal injury is suspected. Slanting the whole patient (such as in the Trendelenburg position) should be avoided if possible, as this causes the abdominal organs to put pressure on the diaphragm, thereby hindering breathing.

10. a. The shock patient's vital signs should be checked every 5 minutes. Although this is not always practical in the field, it should be attempted if possible.

11. d. When managing a patient with obvious external blood loss, the EMT should wear appropriate protective gear as dictated by the circumstances. For example, if minimal bleeding without the risk of splash is encountered, gloves may be all that are needed. However, in the event of severe bleeding, the risk of splashing or spurting is much greater and gloves, eye protection, gown, and mask should be used. Use of protective gear should never be based on the patient's admission of having a communicable disease. All patients must be assumed to pose a risk to the EMTs.

12. c. The sudden loss of 1 liter of blood in an adult patient can cause hypovolemic shock. In children, a loss of 500 cc of blood is serious, as is a loss of 100–200 cc of blood in infants.

13. c. Venous bleeding can be recognized as dark-red blood that flows steadily. This type of bleeding is often easily controlled by direct pressure.

14. a. Arterial bleeding is bright red, and the blood spurts with each heartbeat. This type of bleeding may not be easily controlled and can be rapidly fatal.

15. b. Bleeding from the capillaries is characterized by a slow, oozing flow of dark-red blood. Pressure points are not used to control capillary bleeding.

16. a. Application of direct pressure is the first step in bleeding control. The pressure may be concentrated (such as when a fingertip is used to press on the bleeding point) or diffuse (such as when it is applied over a larger area of injury). Diffuse pressure occludes the arteries and veins that lead to the injury.

17. d. The PASG, the hand, or an air splint may be used to apply direct pressure to a wound. A narrow bandage should not be used, as it applies too much pressure to a narrow area and may impair circulation or damage underlying blood vessels and nerves.

18. d. Elevation of an extremity may supplement direct pressure for bleeding control. Ice should never be placed directly on a wound.

19. c. The brachial artery, located in the upper arm, is the pressure point of choice for controlling bleeding from a forearm injury.

20. d. The femoral artery, located in the groin, is the best pressure point to use to control bleeding from a leg injury.

21. a. Digital pressure should not be used alone. The EMT should continue to apply direct pressure to the wound, as the bleeding area may be supplied by more than one artery. Digital pressure should be applied on the pressure point as close to the wound as possible.

22. b. Tourniquets should be used *only* as a last resort. They are not automatically necessary in cases of amputation or crush injury.

23. a. When a bandage is used as a tourniquet, it should be wrapped twice around an extremity before being tightened. It should be 4 inches wide and six to eight layers deep. The tourniquet is applied proximal to the wound, but as distal on the extremity as possible. It should never be loosened after it is applied, as this will flood the body with acidotic blood.

24. b. Tourniquets must be applied tight enough to occlude arterial blood flow. If only venous blood is occluded, bleeding may become worse because the bleeding site is still supplied with blood but return of venous blood is prevented.

25. a. After applying a tourniquet, document its use and the time it was applied on the EMS report. Some sources advocate writing the letters "TK" and the time the tourniquet was applied on the patient's forehead.

26. d. Blood-pressure cuffs may gradually lose pressure. They are wide enough to be used as tourniquets; however, if used as such they must be monitored constantly for pressure loss. Hemostats may be used to clamp the cuff tubes, potentially reducing pressure loss.

27. **c.** Epistaxis is another term for nosebleed. Epinephrine (also known as adrenalin) is a hormone produced by the adrenal glands, epiphyseal means pertaining to long bones, and epidural means upon the dura.

28. **b.** When managing a nosebleed with no associated spinal injury, the EMT should have the patient lean forward if possible. This helps prevent blood from going down the patient's throat. The EMT may also pinch the fleshy portion of the patient's nostrils together.

29. **c.** When managing a patient with a head injury accompanied by a nosebleed, do not attempt to stop the bleeding, as this can increase pressure in the head. Do not tip the head back, because head injuries may be accompanied by neck injuries, which should be stabilized by appropriate means.

30.
__rib__	125 cc (¼ unit)
__humerus__	250 cc (½ unit)
__tibia__	500–750 cc (1–1½ units)
__femur__	1,000 cc (2 units)
__pelvis__	1,000–10,000 cc (2–20 units)

31. **d.** Internal bleeding of the stomach should be suspected if emesis looks like coffee grounds. This appearance is caused by partial digestion of blood.

32. **c.** Stools that resemble tar indicate internal bleeding in the upper intestines. Bright-red blood may be associated with bleeding lower in the intestines.

33. **b.** Signs of internal bleeding include bright-red blood in the stool or vomitus; an enlarged, tender, rigid abdomen; and signs of hypovolemic shock. The patient may complain of extreme thirst.

34. **c.** If the EMT suspects that the patient has internal bleeding, he or she should be alert for the possibility of subsequent nausea and vomiting.

35. **c.** Bilateral femur fractures may be accompanied by moderate to severe shock due to severe bleeding into the tissues surrounding the fractured area of bone.

36. **a.** A pelvic injury with signs of abdominal bleeding is an indication for use of the PASG. The PASG should not be used if the patient has chest injuries or an isolated head injury.

37. **c.** PASG should not be applied if auscultation reveals sounds indicating fluid in the lungs.

38. **a.** The top of the PASG should lie immediately below the level of the diaphragm.

39. **b.** The PASG should be inflated only after approval is given by medical direction.

40. **c.** The PASG should be inflated until the Velcro™ starts to crackle or the pop-off valves release. Gauges tend to be inaccurate and are not often used. If gauges are used, a pressure of 60 mm Hg is recommended. Always follow your local protocols.

41. **d.** Deflation of the PASG should not be done in the field. It should be accomplished by trained personnel in a clinical setting. Generally, deflation should be stopped after each 5 mm Hg drop in patient blood pressure. The EMT should be familiar with deflation procedures in the event that instruction needs to be given to hospital personnel who are less familiar with the device. Always follow your local protocols for deflation.

CHAPTER 11

SOFT-TISSUE INJURIES

1. When dealing with open soft-tissue injuries, the EMT must remember:
   a. that soft-tissue injuries are generally life-threatening
   b. to pay particular attention to avoiding contact with body substances
   c. bleeding control takes priority over all other care
   d. the injuries are generally worse than they appear

2. An example of a closed soft-tissue injury would be:
   a. an incision
   b. a hematoma
   c. a compound fracture
   d. epistaxis

3. When bruising is noted over the area of a vital organ:
   a. a superficial injury should be suspected
   b. direct pressure should be applied to the area
   c. damage to the underlying organ and internal bleeding should be suspected
   d. it is only of concern if it is noted on the abdomen and not the chest

4. Match the following types of open soft-tissue injuries with their descriptions: **abrasion, amputation, avulsion, laceration, puncture**
   _____ A break in the skin caused by forceful impact with a sharp object. The wound edges may be regular (linear) or irregular (stellate).
   _____ A simple scraping or scratching of the outer layer of the skin. Examples include "rug-burns" or "friction-burns."
   _____ A portion of tissue or skin that is torn loose and left hanging as a flap or is completely pulled from the body.
   _____ A small opening or perforation of the skin typically caused by sharp pointed objects.
   _____ The removal of an appendage (such as an arm) from the body.

 5. A consideration when managing abrasions is that:
   a. bleeding may be severe
   b. they may become infected by foreign matter
   c. pain is usually minimal
   d. sterile dressings are not needed because the wound is not deep

6. Bleeding from a laceration:
   a. is always easy to control
   b. is usually not as severe if wound edges are smooth
   c. may be severe and difficult to control
   d. primarily comes from the capillaries

7. A gunshot wound is classified as a:
   a. laceration
   b. puncture wound
   c. perforating wound
   d. sterile wound

8. Another term for a bruise is:
   a. abrasion
   b. urticaria
   c. hematocrit
   d. contusion

9. A lump at a wound site caused by blood collecting within damaged tissue is a:
   a. hematoma
   b. varicose vein
   c. fistula
   d. melanoma

10. One of the goals of managing an open wound is to:
    a. thoroughly clean the wound before dressing it
    b. remove any clots that have formed prior to the arrival of EMS
    c. provide immediate care
    d. prevent further wound contamination

11. A dressing should do all of the following *except:*
    a. hold a bandage in place
    b. help control bleeding
    c. prevent further contamination and infection
    d. protect the wound from further injury or damage

12. When bandaging an extremity:
    a. place knots over the wound
    b. cover all fingertips and toes to prevent further injury
    c. secure any loose bandage ends
    d. wrap the bandage tightly enough to occlude venous blood flow

 13. If blood soaks through the dressings:
    a. apply fresh dressings over the blood-soaked ones and continue applying pressure
    b. remove all the blood-soaked dressings and apply fresh ones
    c. apply a tourniquet
    d. lower an extremity below the level of the heart

14. When managing an impaled object:
    a. control bleeding by applying pressure on the object
    b. stabilize the object with a bulky dressing
    c. remove the object and apply direct pressure to the wound to control bleeding
    d. never remove the object

15. Examine the patient for an exit wound whenever encountering:
    a. a penetrating or puncture injury
    b. an avulsion
    c. a partial amputation
    d. a stellate laceration

16. Early management of an open chest injury includes:
    a. covering the wound with saline-soaked gauze pads
    b. supporting the injured area with sandbags
    c. sealing the wound with an occlusive dressing
    d. placing the patient on a backboard

17. If no spinal injuries are suspected, a patient with an open chest injury should be placed:
    a. supine with the legs elevated
    b. in a position of comfort
    c. in a prone position
    d. on the right side with the head lower than the legs

18. A critical factor when managing open chest injuries is:
    a. early application of a cervical collar
    b. access to an AED
    c. use of a flow-restricted, oxygen-powered ventilation device
    d. early administration of high-flow oxygen

19. If, after an open chest injury is sealed, the patient becomes cyanotic and dyspnea increases:
   a. place a second, larger occlusive dressing over the first
   b. release the dressing to allow air to escape
   c. turn the victim onto the side opposite the wound
   d. turn down the oxygen to avoid hyperventilation

20. Management of an evisceration includes:
   a. replacing the organ within the abdomen
   b. applying a moist, sterile dressing to the area and covering it with an occlusive dressing
   c. applying direct pressure to the evisceration to control bleeding
   d. applying the PASG and inflating the legs and abdominal compartment

21. The position of choice for a patient with an evisceration and no accompanying spinal or leg injuries is on the:
   a. back with the hips and knees flexed
   b. back with the hips and knees straight
   c. left side
   d. right side

22. An impaled object may need to be removed if it:
   a. interferes with the airway
   b. is lodged in the ear
   c. is too small to be x-rayed
   d. is lodged in the nose

23. If a patient is found with an object impaled through the cheek:
   a. do not remove the object
   b. remove the object by carefully pulling it out in the direction opposite from which it entered
   c. remove the object with a twisting motion
   d. remove the object by carefully pulling it out in the same direction it entered

24. To package an amputated part for transportation to the hospital:
   a. pack it in ice
   b. immerse it in sterile water
   c. wrap it in a sterile dressing and keep it cool
   d. wrap it in a wet, sterile dressing and keep it warm

25. When managing a partial avulsion or amputation:
   a. leave the part in the position found
   b. complete the amputation with sterile scissors
   c. apply direct pressure to the skin flap to control bleeding
   d. gently straighten and align any skin bridges

26. Injuries to the neck or throat:
   a. are classified as closed or blunt
   b. are serious only if they involve open wounds
   c. are classified as open or sharp
   d. should always be considered serious

27. A serious complication associated with an open neck injury is:
   a. air embolism
   b. tracheal deviation
   c. increased blood pressure
   d. neck vein distention

28. Management of an open neck injury may include:
   a. placing the patient in a sitting position
   b. applying digital pressure to a brachial artery
   c. covering the wound with a sterile occlusive dressing
   d. having the patient stand to reduce blood flow through the neck

29. When managing a patient with an injury to the soft tissue of the neck, always suspect:
   a. internal bleeding
   b. accompanying jaw injuries
   c. cervical spine injury
   d. accompanying chest injuries

30. When managing an injured eye:
    a. also cover the uninjured eye
    b. leave the uninjured eye uncovered
    c. apply dry gauze pads to the eye
    d. use a compression dressing

✱ 31. Management of a burned eye or eyelid would include:
    a. leaving both eyes uncovered
    b. covering the eye with dry, sterile dressings
    c. covering both eyes with moist dressings
    d. covering both eyes with gauze dressings coated with petroleum jelly

32. When managing a patient with an impaled object in the eye:
    a. remove the object if it interferes with placement of a metal eye shield
    b. remove the object if transport time to the hospital is longer than 20 minutes
    c. remove the object and apply pressure to the wound
    d. never remove the object

✱ 33. Before applying a metal eye shield:
    a. pad the edges of the eye shield
    b. flush the patient's eye
    c. place an occlusive dressing over the eye
    d. cover the holes with tape

✱ 34. Lacerations of the eyeball can be managed by:
    a. applying direct pressure to the eye
    b. covering the eye with a metal eye shield or protective cup
    c. covering the eye with a gauze pad
    d. irrigating the eye with sterile water

✱ 35. When flushing a patient's eyes:
    a. flush from the outside corner to the inside corner
    b. apply the water in a slow, dripping fashion
    c. flush from the inside corner to the outside corner
    d. irrigate with the eyes closed

36. The major concern when managing a patient with a mouth injury is:
    a. airway compromise
    b. permanent disfigurement
    c. hypoperfusion
    d. swelling of brain tissue

37. Burn injuries are typically classified as any of the following *except:*
    a. chemical
    b. steam
    c. electrical
    d. thermal

38. A burn characterized by reddening, blister formation, and intense pain is a:
    a. full-thickness burn
    b. superficial burn
    c. partial-thickness burn
    d. medium-thickness burn

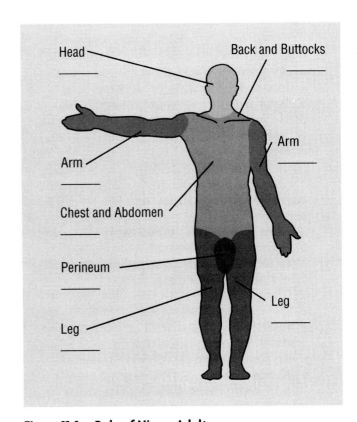

Figure 11-1   Rule of Nines–Adult.

39. Using the given list of percentages, label each part of the adult in Figure 11-1 with the proper percentage of body surface area.
    1%, 9%, 9%, 9%, 18%, 18%, 18%, 18%

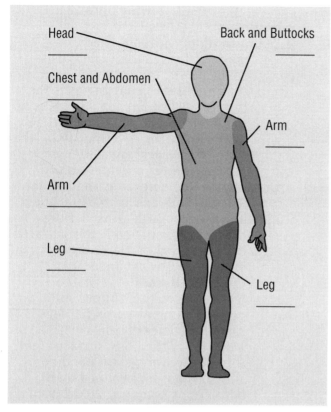

Figure 11-2   Rule of Nines–Child.

 40. Using the given list of percentages, label each part of the 5-year-old child in Figure 11-2 with the proper percentage of body surface area.
9%, 9%, 14%, 16%, 16%, 18%, 18%

41. Using the given list of percentages, label each part of the infant in Figure 11-3 with the proper percentage of body surface area.
9%, 9%, 14%, 14%, 18%, 18%, 18%

For questions 42–44, use the Rule of Nines to calculate the approximate percentage of burns.

42. A 48-year-old man has been injured in a gas heater explosion. He has burns covering his entire right arm, entire back, and the back of his head. You estimate the burns to cover a body surface area of about:
a. 18%
b. 27%
c. 31%
d. 40%

43. A 5-year-old girl has pulled a pot of boiling water off the stove while helping her mother make supper. She has burns on the chest, abdomen, and the front of both legs. You estimate the burns to cover a body surface area of about:
a. 22%
b. 34%
c. 48%
d. 56%

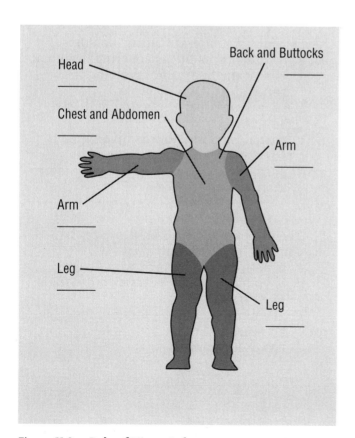

Figure 11-3   Rule of Nines–Infant.

44. An 8-month-old infant has been rescued from a burning house by firefighters. Upon examination, you find that the infant has partial-thickness burns on the buttocks and the back of both legs. You estimate the burns to cover a body surface area of about:
a. 9%
b. 14%
c. 23%
d. 30%

45. Superficial burns involve:
a. only the dermis
b. only the epidermis
c. the epidermis and dermis
d. all layers of the skin

✳ 46. Respiratory tract burns should be suspected if a patient:
a. has singed or sooty nasal hairs, nostrils, or lips
b. has a hoarse voice
c. was in a closed room during a fire
d. all of the above

47. Patients with suspected inhalation injuries:
a. should not be placed on oxygen to avoid drying of the mucous membranes
b. will display signs of respiratory distress within 1 hour of the injury
c. should always be transported to the hospital
d. have a cherry-red color

48. The palm of a patient's hand may be used as a guide when estimating burn percentages of small areas because it represents an area of approximately:
a. 0.5% of body surface
b. 1% of body surface
c. 2% of body surface
d. 3% of body surface

49. Mark each of the following burns as: **minor, moderate, critical**
_____ A timer on a tanning bed malfunctions. Superficial burns cover 85% of the patient.
_____ A weekend mechanic removes the cap from a hot radiator. He manages to protect his face but has partial-thickness burns covering 10% of the front of his chest and abdomen.
_____ A spark ignites a welder's shirt. Workmates quickly extinguish the fire, but full- and partial-thickness burns cover both arms and the chest; 18% of the body surface area has sustained partial-thickness burns and 5% sustained full-thickness burns.
_____ A woman cooking supper spills a pot of boiling water on her legs. Partial-thickness burns cover 18%–20% of the body surface area.
_____ A roofer wearing shorts and no shirt has hot tar dropped on his body. Approximately 20%–24% of the body surface area has partial-thickness burns—one arm is completely encompassed.

50. For adults, moderate burns include:
a. full-thickness burns covering less than 10% of the body and involving the hands, feet, face, or groin
b. superficial burns covering more than 30% of the body
c. partial-thickness burns involving 15%–30% of the body
d. partial-thickness burns covering more than 40% of the body

51. The age of a burn victim is of special concern if the patient:
a. is between 20 and 45 years of age
b. is younger than 5 years or older than 55 years
c. is younger than 10 years or older than 50 years
d. has other injuries

52. A partial-thickness burn in a child is considered moderate if it covers:
    a. 5%–10% of the body
    b. 10%–20% of the body
    c. 20%–30% of the body
    d. 30%–40% of the body

53. Moderate pain with associated redness but no blistering is characteristic of a:
    a. superficial burn
    b. partial-thickness burn
    c. medium-thickness burn
    d. full-thickness burn

54. A burn associated with a painful, swollen deformed extremity would be considered:
    a. minor
    b. moderate, provided that it only involves a lower extremity
    c. moderate, regardless of the extremity involved
    d. critical

55. The first step in managing a burn patient is to:
    a. estimate the percentage of burns
    b. ensure an adequate airway and assess breathing
    c. stop the burning process
    d. apply sterile burn dressings

56. A burn characterized by leathery, dry skin that may appear white or charred and that may be accompanied by little or no pain is a:
    a. superficial burn
    b. partial-thickness burn
    c. medium-thickness burn
    d. full-thickness burn

❋ 57. When caring for burns to the hands or feet:
    a. apply burn cream on each digit
    b. place nothing between the digits
    c. separate each digit with sterile gauze
    d. advanced medical care is usually not needed unless full-thickness burns are present

58. Burn management should include:
    a. applying ice directly to the burn
    b. removing jewelry and smoldering clothing
    c. removing charred clothing stuck to a burn
    d. removing hot tar from a burn

59. Ointments or greases should:
    a. only be used on burns if they are sterile
    b. never be used on burns by EMTs
    c. be applied immediately after the burning process has stopped
    d. only be applied to extremity burns

❋ 60. An important consideration when managing burns is that:
    a. burn patients lose body heat easily
    b. all burn patients should go to the nearest hospital
    c. burn patients are often overheated
    d. there is no risk of hypoperfusion unless other injuries are present

61. When managing a patient with burns caused by a chemical powder:
    a. cover the chemical with a sterile, moist dressing
    b. brush off as much of the chemical as possible
    c. wash the chemical off slowly
    d. cover the chemical with a sterile, dry dressing

62. Irrigate liquid chemical burns to the body:
    a. only with sterile solutions
    b. with a neutralizing solution
    c. for no longer than 15 minutes
    d. with copious amounts of water

63. Chemical burns to the eyes should be irrigated:
    a. with a neutralizing solution
    b. only if it does not interfere with transport
    c. until the patient reaches the hospital
    d. for no longer than 10 minutes

64. When caring for a patient with an electrical burn:
    a. discharge any electricity left in the patient
    b. check for entrance and exit wounds
    c. pull the patient off electrical wires
    d. ascertain the exact voltage that caused the burn

65. Electrical burns differ from other burns in that:
    a. there is no injury from heat
    b. they heal faster than ordinary burns
    c. damage is always limited to the dermis and epidermis
    d. tissue damage may be deeper and more severe than it appears

66. A major problem associated with lightning or electrical burns is:
    a. respiratory and cardiac arrest
    b. abdominal injury
    c. head bleeds
    d. tension pneumothorax

ADDITIONAL POINTS FOR DISCUSSION

1. What are some types of occlusive dressings?

2. If a commercially produced occlusive dressing is not available, what other items carried on the ambulance may be adapted?

3. What are the procedures for notifying local authorities of an animal attack or bite?

4. Where is the nearest rabies control center for your area?

5. Which hospital(s) in your area have the capability of reattaching an amputated limb?

6. What are your local protocols regarding the removal of contact lenses?

7. How would you remove a:

    * Hard contact lens?

    * Soft contact lens?

8. To which hospital(s) in your area would you transport a patient with severe burns?

9. Do your local protocols allow the use of wet dressings? If so, in what cases? What is the maximum amount of body surface that may be covered by wet dressings?

10. To which hospital(s) would you transport a patient with a chemical burn or contamination?

11. What precautions can be taken before transporting to avoid unnecessary contamination of the ambulance and equipment?

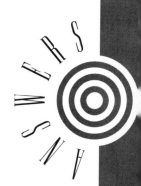

11 SOFT-TISSUE INJURIES

1. **b.** When dealing with open soft-tissue injuries, the EMT should pay particular attention to avoiding contact with body substances. Such precautions include wearing gloves and other personal protective equipment as well as washing the hands as soon as possible after managing the patient. A waterless hand cleaner should be used if running water is not available. Soft-tissue injuries are generally not life-threatening and tend to look much worse than they really are. Ensuring an adequate airway takes priority over controlling bleeding.

2. **b.** A hematoma is an example of a closed soft-tissue injury. A contusion is another example.

3. **c.** When bruising is noted over the area of a vital organ, suspect damage to the underlying organ and possible internal bleeding. Direct pressure does not control internal bleeding. Although the ribs of the chest provide some protection, a blow of enough force to bruise the chest wall can also bruise lung or heart tissue. Although this may not cause internal bleeding as severe as that associated with abdominal organs, the results can be equally devastating.

4.
<u>laceration</u> A break in the skin caused by forceful impact with a sharp object. The wound edges may be regular (linear) or irregular (stellate).

<u>abrasion</u> A simple scraping or scratching of the outer layer of the skin. Examples include "rug-burns" or "friction-burns."

<u>avulsion</u> A portion of tissue or skin that is torn loose and left hanging as a flap or is completely pulled from the body.

<u>puncture</u> A small opening or perforation of the skin typically caused by sharp pointed objects.

<u>amputation</u> The removal of an appendage (such as an arm) from the body.

5. **b.** Abrasions are often contaminated by foreign matter since they are associated with friction between the skin and another object, such as ground or pavement. As a result, risk of infection is increased. Bleeding is usually minor and from the capillary beds. Abrasions may be very painful due to the large surface area involved.

6. **c.** Bleeding from a laceration may be severe and difficult to control depending on location and depth. If the wound edges are regular and smooth, the blood vessels may not constrict and the wound may bleed freely.

7. **b.** Gunshot wounds (and stab wounds) are classified as puncture wounds. For a gunshot wound to be considered a "perforating wound," it must travel through the body, and cause an entrance and exit wound. The notion that gunshot wounds are sterile as a result of the heat of the bullet is false—contamination can occur with bits of clothing and dirt carried into the wound.

8. **d.** A contusion is a bruise and can be managed with cold application. Urticaria are itchy wheals or hives, and a hematocrit measures the volume of red blood cells in a specimen.

9. **a.** A hematoma is a lump caused by blood collecting within damaged tissue. Varicose veins are distended veins, a fistula is an abnormal passage, and a melanoma is a tumor or growth.

10. **d.** Preventing further contamination of the wound is a goal of wound management. Other goals include bleeding control and immobilizing the injured part. Thorough cleaning should not be attempted by the EMT, and clots should not be removed. Although open wounds may be graphic, they should not sidetrack the EMT from checking for more serious, life-threatening injuries.

11. **a.** Dressings help control bleeding, prevent further contamination and infection, and protect the wound from further injury or damage. Dressings are held in place by bandages.

12. **c.** Loose bandage ends should be secured so they do not catch on anything. Do not place knots over wounds, on the skin, or on the patient's back. Bandages should not be so tight that they restrict circulation. Do not cover fingertips or toes as this will make it difficult to check for signs of impaired circulation.

13. **a.** If blood soaks through a dressing, the dressing should not be removed, as this may dislodge a partially formed clot. Additional dressings should be placed over the soaked dressing. However, if too many layers are applied, pressure may be lost and bleeding control will be rendered inadequate. The EMT may consider removing all but the few layers of dressings closest to the wound. Fresh dressings can be applied over these.

14. **b.** Impaled objects should be stabilized with bulky dressings. Do not apply pressure to the object. Although the object is usually left in place, there are exceptions. Long objects may be carefully shortened to facilitate transport.

15. **a.** Whenever a penetrating or puncture injury is encountered, the EMT should check for an exit wound. A stellate laceration has irregular edges.

16. **c.** Early management of an open chest injury includes sealing the wound with an occlusive dressing. This should be accomplished at the same time as the airway step.

17. **b.** If no spinal injuries are suspected, a patient with an open chest injury should be placed in a position of comfort that does not interfere with breathing.

18. **d.** Early administration of high-flow oxygen is critical when managing open chest injuries.

19. **b.** If, after an open chest injury is sealed, the patient becomes cyanotic and dyspnea increases, pressure has probably built up in the chest cavity. The EMT should release the dressing to allow air to escape.

20. b. Eviscerations should be covered with moist, sterile dressings that are then covered with an occlusive dressing. The organs should not be replaced, and direct pressure should not be applied to the area. The abdominal compartment of the PASG should not be inflated over an evisceration.

21. a. If there is no accompanying spinal or leg injuries, transport an evisceration patient on his or her back with the hips and knees flexed.

22. a. An impaled object may need to be removed if it interferes with the airway. An object may also need to be removed is if it interferes with chest compressions or with patient transportation. Objects lodged in the ear or nose should not be removed.

23. d. Objects that perforate the cheek wall should usually be removed, as they may interfere with the airway or become dislodged and obstruct the airway. Remove the object by carefully pulling it out in the same direction it entered. If it cannot easily be removed, stabilize the object and leave it in place.

24. c. An amputated part should be wrapped in a sterile dressing and kept cool. It should not be immersed or soaked in water or allowed to freeze.

25. d. Any skin bridges should be gently straightened and aligned in order to maintain circulation in the partially avulsed or amputated part. Skin bridges may also be used to cover the stump if surgical amputation is necessary. The EMT should never complete an amputation or apply pressure to the skin bridge.

26. d. Injuries to the neck or throat should always be considered serious due to the large number of structures located in such a small area. Neck injuries are often blunt or sharp in nature.

27. a. Air embolism may occur when a large neck vein is lacerated.

28. c. A neck vein laceration should be covered with an occlusive dressing to reduce chances of air embolism. The patient should not stand or sit up because this increases the chances of air embolism.

29. c. The EMT should suspect cervical spine injury when an injury to the soft tissue of the neck is encountered.

30. a. When managing an injured eye, cover both eyes. If the uninjured eye is not covered, the injured eye will move whenever the uninjured eye moves. This is known as sympathetic movement. Do not cover an eye with dry gauze, as this can be irritating and the gauze will absorb eye fluids.

31. c. When burns to the eyes or eyelids are encountered, cover both eyes with moist dressings.

32. d. Objects impaled in the eye should not be removed. Stabilize the object and, if possible, cover it with a cone to protect the protruding object from being accidently displaced. Since both eyes move together, cover the uninjured eye to minimize the chances of eye movement.

33. a. The edges of a metal eye shield should be padded before it is applied.

34. b. A lacerated eye should be covered with a metal eye shield or protective cup. Never apply pressure to a lacerated eye, as this can cause a loss of fluid from inside the eye.

35. **c.** Eyes should be flushed from the corner closest to the nose to the outside corner to avoid contaminating the uninjured eye with the runoff. Flushing both eyes can be accomplished using a nasal cannula attached to intravenous tubing if available.

36. **a.** The EMT must always monitor a patient with a mouth injury for airway compromise. Loose teeth and blood can present problems but may be managed with aggressive suctioning.

37. **b.** Burns may be classified as thermal, chemical, or electrical. Some sources also add radiation burns as a fourth category. A steam burn is a thermal burn.

38. **c.** Partial-thickness burns are characterized by reddening, blister formation, and intense pain.

39.

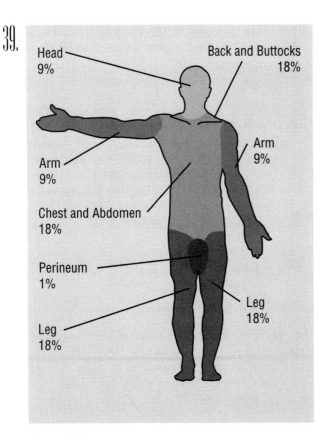

Figure 11-1

40.

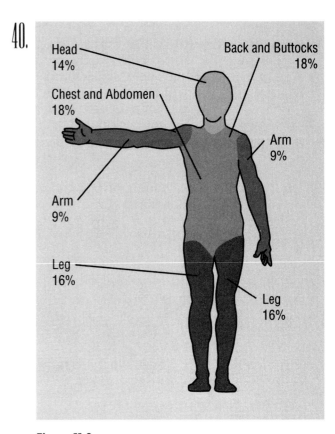

Figure 11-2

41.

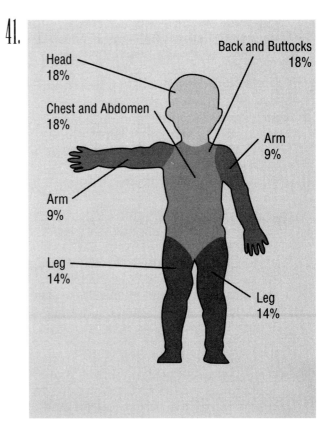

Figure 11-3

42. **c.** The burns cover approximately 31% of body surface area (right arm = 9%, entire back = 18%, back of head = 4%).

43. **b.** Approximately 34% of body surface area is involved (chest and abdomen = 18%, the front of both legs = 16%).

44. **c.** The infant has burns covering approximately 23% of its body (buttocks = 9% and the back of both legs = 14%).

45. **b.** A superficial burn involves only the epidermis. Partial-thickness burns involve the epidermis and part of the dermis. Full-thickness burns involve the full thickness of the skin and may involve underlying muscles, bones, or other structures.

46. **d.** All of the above. Singed or sooty nasal hairs, nostrils, or lips or a hoarse voice are signs of possible respiratory tract burns. Also, respiratory tract burns should be suspected if a patient was in a closed room or confined area that was on fire.

47. **c.** Always transport patients with suspected inhalation injuries to the hospital. The structures of the respiratory tract may swell to the point that the airway becomes occluded.

48. **b.** Generally, the palm of the hand equals approximately 1% of body surface area. This can be helpful when estimating burn percentages of small areas.

49.
moderate A timer on a tanning bed malfunctions. Superficial burns cover 85% of the patient.

minor A weekend mechanic removes the cap from a hot radiator. He manages to protect his face but has partial-thickness burns covering 10% of the front of his chest and abdomen.

critical A spark ignites a welder's shirt. Workmates quickly extinguish the fire, but full- and partial-thickness burns cover both arms and the chest; 18% of the body surface area has sustained partial-thickness burns and 5% has sustained full-thickness burns.

moderate A woman cooking supper spills a pot of boiling water on her legs. Partial-thickness burns cover 18%–20% of the body surface area.

critical A roofer wearing shorts and no shirt has hot tar dropped on his body. Approximately 20%–24% of the body surface has partial-thickness burns—one arm is completely encompassed.

50. **c.** For adults, moderate burns include superficial burns covering more than 50%–75% of the body, partial-thickness burns covering 15%–30% of the body, or full-thickness burns (not involving the face, hands, feet, or genitals) covering 2%–10% of the body.

51. **b.** The age of a burn patient is of special concern if the patient is younger than 5 years or older than 55 years.

52. **b.** In a child, any partial-thickness burn covering 10%–20% of the body is considered moderate. Any full- or partial-thickness burn covering more than 20% of the body is considered critical.

53. **a.** Superficial burns are characterized by redness, moderate pain, and no blister formation.

54. **d.** Burns associated with a painful, swollen, deformed extremity or that involve the respiratory tract are considered critical. They are considered high-priority injuries.

55. **c.** The burning process must be stopped first or the injury process will continue. An open airway and artificial ventilations will do little good if a patient's tissues are still burning.

56. **d.** Full-thickness burns are accompanied by little or no pain due to destruction of nerve endings. The skin may be dry, leathery and white or charred.

57. **c.** When burns of the hands or feet are being dressed, each digit should be separated with a sterile dressing to keep them from sticking together.

58. **b.** Jewelry and smoldering clothing should be removed from the burn area. Clothing that is sticking to the burn should be cooled and left in place to avoid removing the skin. Attempting to remove tar may also cause further tissue injury.

59. **b.** Never use ointments or grease on burns, even if sterile, as they will trap heat in the tissues.

60. **a.** Burn patients lose body heat easily (and quickly) since the skin no longer can function as a heat regulator. The EMT must be alert for this and keep the patient in a warm environment.

61. **b.** Powdered chemicals should be brushed off as much as possible, after which the remaining residue may be washed off with copious amounts of water. A special problem associated with some chemicals is that they react with water.

62. **d.** Liquid chemical burns should be flushed with copious amounts of water. A small amount or trickle may do more harm than good in some cases. The water does not have to be sterile. Neutralizing solutions should be avoided, as these often produce heat as the neutralizing takes place. Continue to flush during the entire transportation process.

63. **c.** Chemical burns to the eyes should be flushed until the patient reaches the hospital. A sterile solution should be used if possible. Eyes should be flushed from the corner closest to the nose to the outside corner to avoid contaminating the uninjured eye with the runoff. Flushing both eyes can be accomplished using a nasal cannula attached to intravenous tubing if available.

64. **b.** Once it is safe to do so, patients who have contacted electrical wires or equipment must be checked for entrance and exit wounds. Electricity does not remain in the patient after removal from the source. If the patient is still in contact with the source, do not touch the patient. Attempt to turn the power off.

65. **d.** Tissue damage caused by electrical burns may be much deeper and more severe than it appears. Electricity readily travels along nerves, blood vessels, and muscles, and is capable of causing severe damage.

66. **a.** Lightning and electrical burns may cause respiratory and cardiac arrest. Although it is not high voltage, 110-volt house current causes most electrocutions because wires and equipment using this voltage are accessible to most people.

CHAPTER 12

MUSCULOSKELETAL INJURIES

1. Two basic groups into which all musculoskeletal injuries may be classified are:
   a. open and closed
   b. deformed and simple
   c. open and compound
   d. simple and angulated

2. The mechanism of injury that causes a musculoskeletal injury may be classified as:
   a. primary or secondary
   b. simple or complex
   c. direct or indirect
   d. lateral or medial

3. Signs and symptoms of an underlying bone or joint injury may include:
   a. pain and deformity
   b. swelling and discoloration
   c. loss of use of an extremity
   d. all of the above

4. The sound or sensation noted when broken bones rub together is known as:
   a. costal grinding
   b. grating
   c. epiphysis
   d. deformity

5. When a patient presents with multiple musculoskeletal injuries and hypoperfusion:
   a. splint all injuries prior to moving the patient to prevent further blood loss
   b. splint only open musculoskeletal injuries prior to moving the patient
   c. perform full body immobilization with a backboard and immediately transport
   d. move the patient to the ambulance cot in whatever manner necessary and transport rapidly

6. Evaluate motor, sensory, and circulatory status of an injured extremity:
   a. before and after splinting
   b. only if there is numbness or loss of sensation below the injury site
   c. only if a deformity is present
   d. only before splinting

7. When properly applied, a splint can:
   a. increase damage to muscles, nerves, and blood vessels
   b. diminish pain
   c. cause a closed injury to become an open injury
   d. all of the above

8. When applied to an injured extremity, the splint should:
   a. immobilize 4 inches above and below the injury
   b. immobilize one joint above and one joint below the injury
   c. be the same length as the bone
   d. be no longer than half the length of the limb

9. To help reduce the swelling that often accompanies musculoskeletal injuries:
   a. massage the injured area
   b. rub ice on the injured area
   c. place the patient in the Trendelenburg position
   d. apply a cold pack to the injured area

10. Reducing blood flow to an injured extremity is best accomplished by:
    a. elevating the extremity
    b. lowering the extremity
    c. applying constricting bands
    d. applying pressure to arterial pressure points

11. If a patient has a severely deformed bone injury and no distal pulses, the limb should:
    a. never be straightened
    b. be realigned while pushing on the limb
    c. be realigned using gentle traction
    d. be splinted with a traction splint

12. If an open musculoskeletal injury with a protruding bone is encountered:
    a. do not try to replace the bone
    b. avoid splinting the limb
    c. use gentle traction to replace the bone
    d. use a traction splint

13. In general, joint injuries should be:
    a. realigned prior to splinting
    b. managed with a traction splint
    c. transported without splinting to save time
    d. splinted in the position found

14. When applying a splint to a joint injury:
    a. straighten the joint to its normal position
    b. wrap the joint with an elastic bandage prior to splinting
    c. immobilize the bones above and below the joint
    d. leave shoes and clothing in place to avoid unnecessary movement of the limb

✱ 15. Serious blood loss may often accompany:
    a. a clavicle injury
    b. an elbow injury
    c. a tibia injury
    d. a femur injury

16. A wire ladder splint is an example of a:
    a. soft splint
    b. rigid splint
    c. lateral splint
    d. trauma splint

17. A vacuum splint is an example of:
    a. a pneumatic splint
    b. an air splint
    c. an arthritic splint
    d. a compound splint

18. A type of splint that can be used to apply pressure to a bleeding area as well as to immobilize an injury is:
    a. a sling and swathe
    b. an air splint
    c. a compound splint
    d. a traction splint

✱ 19. Match the most commonly used type of splint to each injury: (*Note:* More than one type of splint may be appropriate. Include all that apply.)
    pillow, rigid, sling and swathe, traction, vacuum
    _____ mid-femur injury
    _____ ankle injury
    _____ forearm injury
    _____ shoulder injury
    _____ knee injury

20. Before a board splint is used, it should be:
    a. padded
    b. lubricated
    c. powdered
    d. wrapped with plastic or aluminum foil

21. Hand injuries should be splinted:
    a. with the fist clenched
    b. with the fingers outstretched and spread
    c. in the position of function
    d. with the fingers outstretched and together

22. When using a bipolar traction splint to manage a patient with a mid-femur injury, one EMT should begin applying traction:
    a. immediately using manual traction
    b. after sliding the splint under the leg
    c. only if authorized to do so by medical direction
    d. after securing the leg to the splint

23. Before applying the traction splint, the patient's shoe is normally:
    a. left in place
    b. removed
    c. unlaced and left in place
    d. taped to the ankle

24. Application of a bipolar traction splint requires:
    a. one EMT
    b. two EMTs
    c. three EMTs
    d. four EMTs

✱ 25. When moving a patient with a suspected pelvic injury, do *not*:
    a. use the backboard straps
    b. use a scoop stretcher
    c. care for hypoperfusion
    d. log-roll the patient

✱ 26. Pelvic injuries are best immobilized using:
    a. a traction splint
    b. padded board splints
    c. a Thomas half-ring
    d. a PASG and a backboard

27. A complication that may result from applying splints and bandages too tightly is:
    a. angulated joints
    b. a compound deformity
    c. reduced distal circulation
    d. compensatory syndrome

ADDITIONAL POINTS FOR DISCUSSION

1. Review the various types and proper application of splints carried on your ambulance.

2. What type(s) of traction splint does your department carry? Review the proper application of the splint(s).

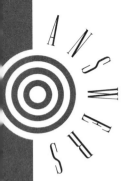

12 MUSCULOSKELETAL INJURIES

1. **a.** Musculoskeletal injuries may be classified as open or closed. Open injuries break the skin and closed injuries do not.

2. **c.** The mechanism of injury associated with musculoskeletal injuries may be classified as direct or indirect. With a direct injury, a force is directly applied to an area of the body and injures that location. With an indirect injury, the force is exerted in one area but the injury occurs in a different location down the bone or at a joint.

3. **d.** All of the above. Signs and symptoms of an underlying bone or joint injury include pain, deformity, swelling, discoloration, loss of use of the extremity or joints locked into place, tenderness, grating, and exposed bone fragments or ends.

4. **b.** The sound or sensation noted when broken bones rub together is known as grating. It is also called crepitus.

5. **c.** Perform a rapid extrication and transport immediately—the backboard can function as a full body splint. When a patient presents with multiple musculoskeletal injuries accompanied by hypoperfusion, time should not be wasted splinting every injury prior to moving.

6. **a.** Evaluate the motor, sensory, and circulatory status of an injured limb before and after splinting.

7. **b.** When properly applied, a splint can diminish pain. Splinting also reduces damage to muscles, nerves, and blood vessels and can prevent a closed injury from becoming an open one.

8. **b.** Splints should immobilize one joint above and one joint below the injury.

9. **d.** A cold pack may be applied to the injured area to help reduce swelling. Do not rub ice directly on the area, as this can cause cold injury to the tissue.

10. **a.** Elevating an injured extremity reduces blood flow to the injured area.

11. **c.** Angulated or deformed bone injuries without distal pulses should be realigned using gentle traction pulled along the long axis of the bone.

12. **a.** Do not try to replace a protruding bone. Apply a sterile dressing over the bone end or open wound.

13. **d.** In general, joint injuries should be splinted in the position found. If circulation is impaired, contact medical direction for advice.

14. c. When applying a splint to a joint injury, the splint should immobilize the bones above and below the joint. Distal pulses should always be checked, and the EMT should be alert for signs of circulatory impairment and bruising. This requires removing shoes and clothing from the injury site.

15. d. A femur injury may be accompanied by serious blood loss into the surrounding tissues. The situation is even more serious if both femurs are injured.

16. b. A wire ladder splint is an example of a rigid splint. Its shape can be formed to the injury. Other examples include padded board splints as well as plastic, metal, or cardboard splints.

17. a. Vacuum splints and air splints are both examples of pneumatic splints.

18. b. Air splints may be used to apply pressure to a bleeding area as well as to immobilize an injury.

19.

_____traction_____	mid-femur injury
___pillow, vacuum___	ankle injury
vacuum, rigid, sling and swathe	forearm injury
___sling and swathe___	shoulder injury
____vacuum, rigid____	knee injury

20. a. Board splints should be padded before they are used.

21. c. Hand (and foot) injuries should be splinted in the position of function.

22. a. When traction to an injured femur is indicated, manual traction should be applied immediately if there are no life-threatening injuries. Do not wait for the traction splint to apply manual traction. Do not use traction splints if the injury is close to the knee or if there is an accompanying injury to the pelvis, hip, knee, lower leg, or ankle. Traction splints should not be used if the patient has a partial amputation with bone separation.

23. b. A patient's shoe should be removed before applying the traction splint. This allows the EMT to check distal pulses and continue to monitor circulatory status after the splint is applied.

24. b. Two EMTs are required to apply a bipolar traction splint. Although only one EMT is needed to apply a unipolar traction splint, it is still preferable to have two EMTs involved. This allows one EMT to manually stabilize the leg while the other applies the splint.

25. d. Patients with suspected pelvic injuries should not be log-rolled. The scoop stretcher or a backboard can be used, and straps should always be used to secure the patient. Pelvic injuries are associated with serious blood loss and shock.

26. d. Pelvic injuries are best immobilized using a PASG and a backboard.

27. c. Reduced distal circulation may result from applying splints and bandages too tightly. If suspected, loosen splints and bandages and reassess.

CHAPTER 13

HEAD AND SPINAL INJURIES

1. When an injured, unconscious patient is encountered, suspect:
   a. a severe allergic reaction
   b. a femur injury
   c. an open chest injury
   d. a spinal injury

2. A mechanism of injury at the scene of a car accident that indiciates a patient may have suffered a traumatic head injury is a:
   a. bent steering column
   b. cracked or deformed windshield
   c. cracked dashboard
   d. broken gearshift lever

3. An indication for applying a cervical collar is:
   a. the patient's history
   b. the patient's signs and symptoms
   c. the mechanism of injury
   d. all of the above

4. Cervical spine immobilization should be accomplished while performing the:
   a. ongoing assessment
   b. focused history
   c. initial assessment
   d. detailed assessment

5. If an injury to the head or spinal cord is suspected:
   a. ask the patient to move his or her head to check for neck pain
   b. check for sensory and motor function in all four extremities
   c. have the patient stand and check for dizziness and pain
   d. check reflexes and capillary refill in all four extremities

6. Adequate cervical spine immobilization may be obtained by:
   a. applying a rigid cervical collar to the patient and sitting the patient in the attendent's chair in the ambulance
   b. using a soft cervical collar, long backboard, and cervical immobilization device
   c. using a rigid cervical collar and a long backboard
   d. any of the above

7. When applying a cervical collar, remember:
   a. to continue to provide manual immobilization until the patient's head can be secured to a backboard
   b. to use whatever size collar is most comfortable for the patient
   c. that all cervical collars are sized the same way
   d. all of the above

8. Rapid extrication is indicated when:
   a. there are other patients with minor injuries in the vehicle who also need extrication
   b. the patient's condition is unstable
   c. the EMT prefers not to use other methods for moving the patient
   d. only two EMTs are available to move the patient

9. Log-rolling the patient should be directed by the:
   a. EMT at the patient's waist
   b. EMT at the patient's shoulders
   c. EMT controlling the patient's head
   d. senior EMS officer

10. If only two EMTs are available to perform a log-roll, one EMT should be positioned:
    a. at the patient's head and the other at the patient's torso
    b. at the patient's shoulders and the other at the patient's hips
    c. at the patient's head and the other at the patient's legs
    d. at the patient's torso and the other slides the board under the patient

11. During the log-roll:
    a. check sensory and motor function in all extremities
    b. apply a cervical collar to the patient
    c. reassess patient vital signs
    d. assess the patient's posterior

12. If a standing patient complains of neck and back pain but is able to walk:
    a. there really is no spinal injury
    b. place the backboard on the cot next to the patient and have the patient lie down on the backboard
    c. apply a short backboard and walk the patient to the cot
    d. immobilize the patient to the backboard while the patient is standing

13. Secure the patient's head to a long backboard:
    a. before applying any backboard straps
    b. after immobilizing the patient's torso to the board
    c. before immobilizing the patient's torso to the board
    d. after securing the patient's legs to the board

14. If voids are encountered between the long backboard and the patient's head and torso:
    a. gently push the patient to conform to the long backboard
    b. remove the patient from the long backboard and use the cot mattress for support
    c. place a pad between the patient and the long backboard
    d. ignore the voids because manipulating the patient may cause further spinal injury

15. If a patient who is secured to a long backboard vomits:
    a. turn the patient's head to one side
    b. roll the secured patient and board to one side as a unit
    c. release the straps and sit the patient up
    d. leave the patient in a supine position and attempt to suction

16. After removing a patient from a vehicle using a rigid shortboard or a vest-type extrication device, the patient should be:
    a. placed flat on an ambulance cot without a backboard
    b. removed from the device and then placed on a long backboard
    c. left in the device and placed on an ambulance cot in a sitting position
    d. left in the extrication device and immobilized to a long backboard

17. When dealing with infants and children with spinal injuries:
   a. place padding from the shoulders to the heels if necessary to provide proper immobilization
   b. do not use a long backboard for immobilization
   c. do not immobilize the patient if it causes excessive restlessness and agitation
   d. do not secure the patient's head to the board

18. Bleeding from scalp injuries:
   a. always indicates a more severe underlying head injury
   b. is very easy to control
   c. normally is arterial
   d. often looks worse than it is

19. Managing scalp injuries should include all of the following *except:*
   a. controlling bleeding
   b. applying a sterile dressing over the wound
   c. cleaning and irrigating the wound
   d. leaving dirt or glass fragments in place

20. The best indicator that a patient has a brain injury is:
   a. altered mental status
   b. increased pulse
   c. decreased breathing
   d. constricted pupils

21. Injury or damage to brain tissue may cause:
   a. a decreased need for oxygen
   b. an increase in pressure inside the skull
   c. a gradual constricting of both pupils
   d. a temporary decrease in brain size

22. A significant sign of skull injury is:
   a. distended neck veins
   b. regular breathing patterns
   c. pale skin
   d. bruising around the eyes or behind the ears

23. When a patient with a traumatic head injury accompanied by low blood pressure and a rapid pulse rate is encountered:
   a. position the patient on the right side with the head lower than the feet
   b. place the patient in a sitting position
   c. suspect other injuries or bleeding
   d. suspect a diabetic emergency

24. Check the level of consciousness of an unstable patient with a head injury:
   a. every 5 minutes
   b. only if a change in mental status is noted
   c. every 15 minutes
   d. only if the vital signs change

25. Concerning unequal pupils, remember that:
   a. unequal pupils are an early sign of head injury
   b. medications do not affect pupils
   c. unequal pupils always indicate a severe head injury
   d. some individuals normally have unequal pupils

26. If a patient with a head injury is bleeding from the nose or ears, be alert for the presence of:
   a. lymph
   b. mucus
   c. cerebrospinal fluid
   d. saline fluid

27. To control bleeding from an open or depressed skull injury:
   a. use a loose, bulky dressing
   b. apply pressure to the injury site
   c. apply digital pressure to the carotid arteries
   d. pack the wound with gauze

28. When managing a patient with a head injury:
   a. also suspect a neck injury
   b. have the patient move his or her head to check for neck pain
   c. do not be concerned unless pupils are unequal
   d. apply a cervical collar and transport the patient sitting upright

29. A patient with a head injury may quickly develop:
   a. an increased level of consciousness
   b. chest pain
   c. nausea and vomiting
   d. hyperglycemia

30. Nontraumatic brain injuries may be a result of:
   a. breathing problems
   b. hemorrhaging or clots
   c. general weakness
   d. altered mental status

31. A patient with a medical or nontraumatic brain injury should be positioned:
   a. on the right side with the head lower than the feet
   b. prone
   c. in the shock position
   d. on the left side

* 32. The best way to reduce brain swelling caused by a head injury is to:
   a. hyperventilate the patient
   b. place the patient on oxygen
   c. place the patient in the Trendelenburg position
   d. apply the PASG

33. Carefully remove a motorcycle or football helmet from a patient if it:
   a. fits the patient's head well
   b. does not have a chin strap
   c. interferes with the airway
   d. does not have a visor

34. The most critical factor when removing a helmet is:
   a. monitoring the pulse for changes
   b. maintaining good cervical spine control
   c. leaving eyeglasses in place
   d. minimizing damage to the helmet

35. Proper removal of a helmet requires at least:
   a. one EMT
   b. two EMTs
   c. three EMTs
   d. four EMTs

ADDITIONAL POINTS FOR DISCUSSION

1. Review the suggested local protocols regarding the appropriate circumstances for the removal of a motorcycle or football helmut.

2. Review the suggested local protocols for removing a helmet from a patient's head.

3. Review the types and proper use of the following spinal immobilization equipment used by your department:

   * Cervical collars:

   * Extrication devices:

   * Head blocks/cervical immobilization devices:

4. What locations (such as buildings or industrial complexes) in your territory may require special packaging and removal techniques for patients?

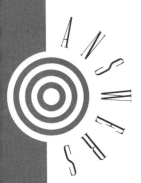

13 HEAD AND SPINAL INJURIES

1. **d.** Suspect spinal injury when managing an injured, unconscious patient. Although physical signs of spinal injury may not be present, be alert for such injury.

2. **b.** Suspect traumatic head injury if a cracked or deformed windshield is noted. A "spiderweb" pattern is typically seen where the patient's head struck the windshield.

3. **d.** All of the above. A cervical collar should be used based on the history, patient signs and symptoms, and mechanism of injury.

4. **c.** Cervical spine immobilization should be accomplished while performing the initial assessment.

5. **b.** A patient with a suspected injury to the head or spinal cord should have sensory and motor function checked in all four extremities. The patient should not be asked to stand, and the neck should not be moved.

6. **c.** A rigid cervical collar and a long backboard (or scoop stretcher) must be used for adequate immobilization of the cervical spine in the field. In addition, head blocks should also be used if available. Soft cervical collars are not acceptable immobilization devices in the field.

7. **a.** Even after a cervical collar is applied, maintain manual immobilization until the patient can be secured to a backboard. There are a variety of sizes of collars available from many manufacturers. The proper size collar should be used. Follow the manufacturer's instructions on choosing the proper size collar for each patient.

8. **b.** Rapid extrication is indicated when the patient is unstable and needs to be immediately moved and transported, or when the scene is unsafe. It may also be used if a patient with less serious injuries is blocking access to a more seriously injured patient. Rapid extrication should not be performed simply because the EMT prefers to move the patient in this method. The number of EMTs present should not be a factor. Other rescue personnel or bystanders may be used to assist extrication regardless of whether it is done rapidly.

9. **c.** The EMT controlling the head directs the log-rolling operation.

10. **a.** If only two EMTs are available to perform a log-roll, one EMT controls the patient's head and neck and the other should be positioned at the patient's torso to control the shoulders and hips.

11. **d.** The patient's entire posterior, or back, should be assessed when the patient is rolled. A cervical collar should already be in place. Sensory and motor function as well as vital signs can be reassessed after the patient is secured to the board.

12. d. A standing patient who is complaining of neck and back pain should be backboarded while standing. A patient's ability to walk does not indicate that no spinal injury exists.

13. b. Secure the patient's head to the long backboard after the torso has been immobilized to the board. Secure the legs to the board after the torso and head are immobilized.

14. c. Pads should be placed to fill voids between the long backboard and the patient's head and torso to prevent any movement. This should be done carefully and in a manner that does not move the patient unnecessarily.

15. b. If a patient is properly secured to a long backboard and begins to vomit, roll the board and the patient to one side as a unit. Patients should not sit up, and their heads should not be turned to the side.

16. d. After a patient is removed from a vehicle using a rigid shortboard or vest-type extrication device, immobilize the patient to a long backboard while he or she is still in the device.

17. a. When immobilizing infants and children, place padding from the shoulders to the heels to fill voids under the patient because a child's head is normally larger in proportion to the size of the body than an adult's. The patient should still be secured to the board. A variety of devices may be used, such as a longboard, shortboard, commercial immobilization device, or padded board splint. Use the device that is the most appropriate for the size of the child. Do not neglect proper immobilization simply because it agitates the patient.

18. d. Bleeding from scalp injuries often looks worse than it is and is not always accompanied by a more severe underlying head injury. The bleeding usually comes from the capillaries but may be difficult to stop because of the number of vessels involved.

19. c. Scalp injuries should not be cleaned or irrigated, as this may force foreign matter into the brain tissue if an underlying skull fracture is present. A loose, bulky sterile dressing can be applied to control bleeding.

20. a. Altered or decreasing mental status should alert the EMT to the presence of a head injury.

21. b. Brain damage or injury may cause an increase in pressure inside the skull.

22. d. Bruising around the patient's eyes or behind the ears is a significant sign of skull injury.

23. c. A patient with a head injury who presents with low blood pressure and a rapid pulse rate probably has other injuries or bleeding. Isolated head injuries do not cause low blood pressure in the early stages.

24. a. Check the level of consciousness of an unstable patient with a head injury every 5 minutes. Any change, whether good or bad, should be noted.

25. d. Remember that some individuals normally have unequal pupils. Caused by increased pressure on the optic nerve, unequal pupils are usually a late sign of head injury. Although they may indicate a serious head injury in an unresponsive patient, unequal pupils alone do not always signify head injury. Medications can also affect pupil size and reactivity.

26. c. Be alert for the presence of cerebrospinal fluid mixed with blood that is discharged from the nose or ears.

27. a. Use a loose, bulky dressing to control bleeding from an open or depressed skull injury. Do not pack the wound or apply pressure to the injury site.

28. a. Always suspect a neck injury when managing a patient with a head injury.

29. c. Increasing pressure inside the head can cause nausea and vomiting. The patient's level of consciousness will decrease.

30. b. Hemorrhaging or clots within the head can cause nontraumatic brain injury.

31. d. Position a patient with a medical or nontraumatic brain injury on the left side to help keep the airway clear.

32. a. Hyperventilating a patient with a head injury can help reduce brain swelling. Placing the patient on oxygen is important, but in itself is not enough to reduce brain swelling. Hyperventilation is needed since it removes carbon dioxide from the system, an important factor in reducing brain tissue swelling.

33. c. The general rule of thumb is that if a helmet interferes with airway control or is loose to the extent that cervical spine immobilization cannot be accomplished, it should be removed. Local protocols concerning removal of helmets should be followed.

34. b. The most critical factor when removing a helmet is maintaining good cervical spine control, which can be difficult. Practice is necessary to develop this skill.

35. b. Proper removal of a helmet requires at least two EMTs.

INFANTS AND CHILDREN

1. Managing infants and children is different from managing adults because younger patients:
   a. are more trustful and less fearful
   b. like to ride in ambulances
   c. tend to be more fearful and may have difficulty communicating
   d. have less difficulty communicating

2. When an infant or child with a non–life-threatening problem is encountered:
   a. take slightly more time to perform the exam
   b. think of the infant or child as a small adult
   c. do not waste time assessing the patient
   d. perform the exam the same way it would be performed on an adult

3. If a procedure is performed that may cause pain:
   a. restrain the child before proceeding
   b. tell the child that it will not hurt
   c. tell the child in advance that it will hurt
   d. have the parents leave the room

4. When caring for a sick or injured child:
   a. never allow parents to be present
   b. allow parents to be present only if absolutely necessary
   c. allow only one parent to be present at any time
   d. make judicious use of the parents for assistance

5. The first concern when assessing an infant or child is:
   a. breathing status
   b. pulse and blood pressure
   c. amount of movement
   d. response to external stimuli

6. An important consideration when managing a sick or injured infant or child is:
   a. the EMT's overall impression of the child's well-being
   b. whether the child has good blood pressure
   c. how many brothers and sisters the child has
   d. that both parents are present before care is begun

7. When performing a detailed physical exam on a newborn or infant, first examine the:
   a. head
   b. neck
   c. abdomen
   d. heart and lungs

8. When performing a detailed physical exam on a toddler:
   a. start with vital signs
   b. use a trunk-to-head approach
   c. examine only exposed areas
   d. use a head-to-toe approach

9. The number one cause of death among infants and children is:
   a. traumatic injury
   b. poisoning
   c. drowning
   d. child abuse

10. When opening the airway of an infant or child:
    a. tilt the head forward
    b. keep the neck totally neutral
    c. tilt the head as far back as possible
    d. do not hyperextend the neck

* 11. An important consideration when caring for infants is that they:
    a. are obligate mouth breathers
    b. are obligate nose breathers
    c. breathe through both the mouth and nose
    d. breathe slower than adults

12. If a child is breathing rapidly and displays signs of increased breathing effort:
    a. respiratory or general fatigue may rapidly develop
    b. the child is simply reacting normally to a stressful situation
    c. immediately assist with a prescribed inhaler
    d. use caution administering oxygen, as it can cause respiratory arrest

13. To insert an oral airway in children:
    a. insert the airway right-side up without using the rotating maneuver that would be used in an adult
    b. the EMT must receive a physician's order for its use
    c. insert the airway upside-down and rotate it once in the proper position
    d. oral airways should not be used on infants or children

14. For newborns with breathing problems:
    a. the use of oxygen is optional
    b. oxygen should be used only if CPR is necessary
    c. the use of oxygen should be avoided, as it will cause blindness
    d. oxygen should be carefully administered

15. If a seriously ill or injured infant or child will not tolerate an oxygen mask:
    a. restrain the child and force him or her to wear the mask
    b. use a blow-by technique to enrich the surrounding air
    c. wait for the child to become unconscious, then administer oxygen
    d. refrain from using oxygen because the hospital will administer it

16. The best way to determine the breathing rate of a newborn or infant is to:
    a. watch the chest rise from a distance
    b. listen with a stethoscope
    c. place one hand on the patient's chest
    d. place one hand on the patient's abdomen

17. The best place to look for cyanosis in an infant or child is the:
    a. lips
    b. belly
    c. eyes
    d. feet

* 18. The pulse rate of infants and children is normally:
    a. slower than that of an adult
    b. faster than that of an adult
    c. the same as that of an adult
    d. weak and thready

* 19. The single most important factor in accurately obtaining a child's blood pressure is the:
    a. child's emotional state
    b. limb used
    c. age of the patient
    d. size of the cuff

20. Blood pressure should be assessed:
    a. only on children younger than 6 years
    b. on all infants and children
    c. only on children older than 3 years
    d. only on children who have sustained trauma

21. A sign of an upper airway obstruction is:
    a. stridor on inspiration
    b. wheezing on expiration
    c. rattling in the chest
    d. rales and rhonchi

22. Lower airway disease should be suspected if the EMT notes:
    a. stridor on inspiration
    b. wheezing on expiration
    c. a slow breathing rate
    d. a sore throat

23. The point at which an infant or child is considered to be in respiratory arrest is when the breathing rate drops below:
    a. 8 breaths per minute
    b. 10 breaths per minute
    c. 12 breaths per minute
    d. 14 breaths per minute

24. Oxygen should be given to infants and children:
    a. only if trauma is present
    b. only if the child will tolerate it
    c. anytime a breathing emergency is present
    d. whenever a child has a breathing rate over 16

25. Febrile seizures:
    a. seldom need evaluation at a hospital
    b. occur in most infants with fevers
    c. signify permanent brain damage
    d. should be considered life-threatening

26. If a child with a history of seizures has just had a seizure, an important question is whether the child:
    a. is following a normal seizure pattern
    b. is taking antiemetic medications
    c. is nauseated or vomiting
    d. all of the above

27. When a child accidently ingests poison:
    a. administer glucose if he or she is semiresponsive
    b. there is no need for transport if the child does not appear to be in distress
    c. make the patient vomit
    d. administer activated charcoal

28. A fever is of particular concern if the child also:
    a. is tired
    b. has a rash
    c. feels achy
    d. cries when being examined

29. Vomiting and diarrhea may be of special concern in children because:
    a. children can dehydrate rapidly
    b. these signs indicate an underlying serious illness
    c. these signs are linked to febrile seizures
    d. children must be given intravenous fluids when these signs occur

30. Blood loss is more significant in children because:
    a. there is less circulating volume
    b. they are difficult to type and crossmatch
    c. the normal clotting factors are not present
    d. the PASG cannot be used on children

31. A sign of hypoperfusion in infants is:
    a. large amounts of tears when crying
    b. decreased urine output
    c. frequent urination
    d. flushed skin

32. Secondary drowning syndrome refers to:
    a. drowning after being injured in the water
    b. drowning after developing respiratory arrest
    c. a medical condition wherein the patient drowns from fluid in the lungs
    d. deterioration that occurs following a near-drowning event and after the patient has resumed normal breathing

33. The cause of sudden infant death syndrome (SIDS) is:
    a. external suffocation
    b. largely unknown
    c. choking
    d. parental neglect

34. When a SIDS situation is encountered:
a. question the parents regarding what they may have done to contribute to the death
b. never institute CPR, as this may compromise the police investigation of the death
c. consider the parents also as patients
d. try to forget about the situation and do not discuss it with other crew members

35. The most common type of trauma in children is:
a. open injury
b. crush injury
c. deceleration injury
d. blunt injury

36. Blood loss in a child is considered serious if the amount exceeds:
a. 5% of total blood volume
b. ½ a unit
c. 500 cc
d. 1 cup

✳ 37. The most accurate indicator of early shock in an infant or child with trauma is:
a. blood pressure
b. pale, cool, and clammy skin
c. a pulse rate greater than 120 beats per minute
d. capillary refill time

38. When a child is a restrained passenger in a motor vehicle accident, suspect:
a. abdominal and lower spinal injuries
b. head injuries
c. chest and arm injuries
d. leg injuries

39. A correct statement concerning PASG use on children is that it should be used:
a. if the patient can be placed in a leg of the garment
b. anytime hypoperfusion is present
c. only if the child fits properly in the garment
d. anytime the blood pressure is below 90 systolic

40. When using the PASG on children, inflate the:
a. legs and then the abdominal compartment
b. abdominal compartment and then the legs
c. abdominal compartment only
d. legs only

41. Physical abuse of a child may be defined as:
a. giving insufficient attention
b. improper or excessive action that injures or causes harm
c. striking as a form of discipline
d. all of the above

42. Suspect child abuse if:
a. an isolated bruise in the process of healing is noted
b. an injury is inconsistent with its described mechanism
c. an isolated scar from a burn is found while examining the patient
d. the parents tell the same story about how the injury occurred

43. If child abuse is suspected:
a. privately report suspicions to the emergency department staff
b. attempt to get the parents to confess to child abuse
c. tell the parents you are going to have them investigated for child abuse
d. take the child to the hospital without parental consent

44. When a child on a home ventilator is encountered:
a. refer to the instruction manual to determine how to operate the unit
b. remove the patient from the ventilator and place him or her on a nonrebreather mask at 15 lpm
c. have the parents assist in managing the patient
d. start CPR and transport

45. If bleeding is noted in the area of a central IV line:
   a. soak up the blood with loose, bulky dressings
   b. apply ice to the area
   c. clamp off the IV tubing
   d. control the bleeding by applying pressure

46. A gastrostomy tube:
   a. hooks directly into a major blood vessel
   b. is placed directly into the brain to relieve intracranial pressure
   c. is placed directly into the trachea through a hole in the neck
   d. is placed directly into the stomach for feeding

47. Two positions in which an infant or child with a gastrostomy tube may be transported are:
   a. lying on the back, or lying on the left side with the head lower than the trunk
   b. sitting, or lying on the right side with the head elevated
   c. in a position of comfort, or prone with the head lower than the trunk
   d. supine, or prone with the head elevated

48. A shunt runs from:
   a. the brain to the abdomen to drain excess cerebrospinal fluid
   b. the heart to the lungs to reoxygenate blood
   c. the ears to the throat to relieve pressure behind the eardrum
   d. the kidneys to the bladder to drain excess urine

49. Infants or children with shunts are particularly prone to:
   a. high fevers
   b. rapid heart rates
   c. respiratory arrest
   d. hypoperfusion

ADDITIONAL POINTS FOR DISCUSSION

1. What are your local and state laws regarding reporting suspected cases of child abuse?

2. What are your local protocols regarding the handling of a SIDS situation?

3. Is there a SIDS crisis group in your area? If so, how can they be contacted?

4. What hospital(s) in your area are able to handle a child with severe trauma?

5. Are there any children within your response area with medical problems who are receiving special medical care at home? If so, what type of medical problem is it? What type of care is being provided? Is there anything that would need to be done differently when responding to an EMS call on these patients?

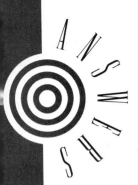

14 INFANTS AND CHILDREN

1. **c.** Infants and children tend to be more fearful than adults and may have difficulty communicating. The ambulance may present a frightening environment for a child.

2. **a.** Unless a serious emergency exists, take a little more time when dealing with a child to explain and perform the exam. This will help put the child at ease. Alter the exam to fit the circumstances but do not skip the assessment. Infants and children should not be thought of as "little adults."

3. **c.** Tell a child in advance if a procedure will hurt. If a child is lied to or surprised, he or she may not trust the EMT for the remainder of the care period. Parents can be used to lend support provided they can handle the situation. Do not restrain a child unless absolutely necessary.

4. **d.** Make judicious use of the parents to assist in examining and caring for infants and children. Parents can be used to calm the child. If a parent is agitated, however, this will agitate the child.

5. **a.** When assessing a child, the first concern is the patient's breathing status. This is especially important with young children and infants, as cardiac arrest is normally secondary to respiratory arrest. Aggressive airway management can make a difference.

6. **a.** The EMT's overall impression of the child's well-being is an important consideration. Physical signs may not always be as valuable as the EMT's impression of how serious the child's injuries are. Although it is best to have the permission of one parent in order to institute care for a child, care can be rendered under implied consent if no parents are present.

7. **d.** When performing a detailed physical exam on a newborn or infant, examine the heart and lungs first and the head last. It is best to obtain heart and lung sounds before the child becomes agitated by the rest of the exam.

8. **b.** When performing a detailed physical exam on a toddler, use a trunk-to-head approach. This approach is used to build confidence and should be taken before the child becomes agitated. Airway, breathing, and circulation still take priority over vital signs.

9. **a.** Traumatic injury is the number one cause of death among infants and children.

10. **d.** When opening the airway of an infant or child, do not hyperextend the neck. Hyperextending the neck can cause airway obstruction.

11. b. Infants are obligate nose breathers. In many cases, suctioning the secretions from an infant's nasopharynx can improve breathing problems.

12. a. A child who is breathing rapidly and displays signs of increased breathing effort is compensating. The child's condition may deteriorate quickly due to rapid respiratory muscle fatigue or general fatigue.

13. a. Oral airways are inserted differently in children than in adults. Because of loose teeth and soft tissue, the airway should be inserted right-side up and not upside-down and rotated. A tongue blade should be used to assist in placement.

14. d. Oxygen should be carefully administered to newborns with breathing problems. Local medical protocols should be followed regarding the exact means for administering oxygen to both newborns and infants. In most cases, oxygen can be carefully administered via a nonrebreather mask or through use of a blow-by method where appropriate. Avoid directing the oxygen at the infant's face, as this can irritate the trigeminal nerve and cause the baby to stop breathing. This situation can be minimized by using warm oxygen and directing the flow to one side of the baby's nose.

15. b. If a seriously ill or injured infant or child will not tolerate an oxygen mask, use a blow-by technique. This can be accomplished using a variety of methods. Oxygen tubing can be held about 2 inches from the patient's face, or it may be inserted into a paper cup held near the child's face. As an alternative, an oxygen mask may be held near the child's face. The objective is to increase the concentration of oxygen in the surrounding air. A good indication of the child's need for oxygen is whether he or she will accept it. Seriously ill or injured infants or children do not usually fight the oxygen mask.

16. a. The best way to determine the breathing rate of a newborn or infant is to watch the chest rise from a distance. Touching the child can cause agitation that will affect the breathing rate.

17. a. The best place to look for cyanosis in an infant or child is the lips or the tongue. Use caution if checking the nail beds of an infant—even when they appear cyanotic, they still may not be an accurate indicator of central circulation status.

18. b. The pulse rate of infants and children is normally faster than that of adults because of the faster metabolic rate.

19. d. The single most important factor in accurately obtaining a child's blood pressure is the size of the cuff.

20. c. Blood pressure should only be assessed on children older than 3 years.

21. a. Stridor heard on inspiration is a sign of upper airway obstruction.

22. b. If the EMT notes wheezing on expiration, lower airway disease should be suspected.

23. b. An infant or child is considered to be in respiratory arrest when the breathing rate drops below 10 breaths per minute. The patient may also exhibit lack of muscle tone, unconsciousness, slow or absent heart rate, and weak or absent distal pulses. Artificial ventilation should be started immediately.

24. c. Anytime a breathing emergency is present, administer oxygen.

25. **d.** Febrile seizures should be considered life-threatening. They usually occur in children 6 months to 5 years of age and are generalized seizures. Approximately 5% of children with fevers develop febrile seizures, but most never have a repeat episode. The child should be evaluated at a hospital.

26. **a.** If a child with a history of seizures has just experienced a seizure, determine if the seizure is similar to others the child has experienced or if anything is different. Also ask if the child is on antiseizure medication.

27. **d.** When a child ingests poison, contact medical direction concerning whether to administer activated charcoal. The patient should be assessed at a hospital, as the effects of some poisons may not be seen for some time after the ingestion.

28. **b.** Fever accompanied by a rash may indicate a serious situation.

29. **a.** Vomiting and diarrhea can cause rapid dehydration in infants and children. These signs do not always indicate serious illness (gastrointestinal upset may even accompany an ear infection). Administration of intravenous fluids is not always necessary.

30. **a.** Since children have less circulating blood volume, a loss of what seems to be even a small amount of blood may lead to shock.

31. **b.** Decreased urine output is a sign of hypoperfusion in infants. To determine if this sign is present, ask parents about diaper wetting. The patient will be pale, and tears will be absent even when the child is crying.

32. **d.** Secondary drowning syndrome refers to deterioration that occurs following a near-drowning event and after the patient resumes normal breathing. This syndrome may occur minutes or hours later.

33. **b.** The cause of sudden infant death syndrome (SIDS) is largely unknown.

34. **c.** Parents of SIDS babies should be viewed as patients also. Do not question them on what they may have done to contribute to the death, as there are usually no external factors involved. They will already feel guilty, and questioning will add to the guilt. CPR may be initiated, and the child may be transported if the parents desire. The situation may be very stressful to the EMT as well, and should be discussed if the crew wishes.

35. **d.** Blunt injury is the leading cause of traumatic death in children.

36. **c.** Blood loss exceeding 500 cc in a child is considered serious.

37. **d.** Delayed capillary refill time is the most accurate indicator of shock in infants and children. Adequate blood pressure in children can often be maintained until the end, and tends to drop only immediately before death.

38. **a.** When a child is a restrained passenger in a motor vehicle accident, suspect abdominal and lower spinal injuries. With children, lap belts are often improperly positioned above the pelvis. In an accident, compression injuries to the soft abdominal organs can occur. If the child is not wearing a shoulder strap, the uncontrolled forward movement of the upper body can cause spinal injuries.

39. **c.** Use the PASG on children only if the child fits properly in the garment. Do not place the child in one leg of the garment. The device may be used in cases of trauma with signs of severe hypotension and pelvic instability. Follow your local protocols on indications for use.

40. d. When using the PASG on children, inflate the legs only—do not inflate the abdominal compartment because children use their abdominal muscles for breathing. The younger the child, the more he or she uses these muscles to breathe. Inflation of the abdominal compartment can greatly interfere with the child's breathing. Consult local protocols for precise guidelines on inflating the PASG for children.

41. b. Physical abuse of a child is improper or excessive action that injures or causes harm. Giving insufficient attention to a child is considered neglect. Physical abuse and neglect are the two forms of child abuse an EMT is likely to encounter.

42. b. Suspect child abuse if the injury is inconsistent with its described mechanism or if the parents cannot account for all the child's injuries. If the child displays different injuries, such as burns or bruises in various stages of healing, this should also alert the EMT to the possibility of child abuse. Repeated calls to the same residence or for the same child to provide care for various injuries may also be a clue. An isolated injury or burn does not necessarily signal abuse.

43. a. If child abuse is suspected, report it privately to the emergency department staff. It should also be reported to the appropriate authorities as specified by state and local laws. Do not discuss it with the parents. Parental consent normally must still be obtained before a child can be transported.

44. c. When a child on a home ventilator is encountered, have the parents assist in managing the patient since they should be familiar with the operation of the ventilator. Do not remove the patient from the ventilator since it is breathing for the patient. If the ventilator malfunctions, manually ventilate the patient.

45. d. If bleeding is noted in the area of a central IV line, control the bleeding by applying pressure. Do not apply ice to the area or clamp off the IV tubing.

46. d. A gastrostomy tube is placed directly into the stomach for feeding.

47. b. Two positions in which an infant or child with a gastrostomy tube may be transported are sitting, or lying on the right side with the head elevated.

48. a. A shunt runs from the brain to the abdomen to drain excess cerebrospinal fluid.

49. c. Infants and children with shunts are particularly prone to respiratory arrest.

CHAPTER 15

MISCELLANEOUS

LEGAL ISSUES

1. A contractual or legal obligation that requires an EMT to provide emergency medical care is a:
   a. good Samaritan act
   b. medico-ethical act
   c. statute to act
   d. duty to act

2. Deviating from the accepted standard of care that a reasonable, prudent EMT would render is:
   a. abandonment
   b. breach of contract
   c. negligence
   d. breach of duty

3. Assistance may be rendered to an unconscious patient or to an ill child whose parents or guardians cannot be reached under the law of:
   a. actual consent
   b. informed consent
   c. implied consent
   d. minor's consent

4. Terminating care of a patient without assuring continuation of care at the same level or higher, or without the patient's consent to stop rendering care is:
   a. breach of contract
   b. assault and battery
   c. breach of consent
   d. abandonment

5. The four components necessary to prove negligence are:
   a. duty to act, breach of duty, injury, and proximate cause
   b. actual consent, breach of duty, damage, and breach of confidentiality
   c. duty to act, breach of contract, injury, and abandonment
   d. lack of informed consent, duty to act, breach of contract, and damage

6. An EMS report or record:
   a. should be thorough and accurate
   b. is not important if the EMT has a good memory
   c. is of little value if an EMT is sued
   d. cannot be used in court

7. EMT guidelines that are established by local and state laws or protocols, professional organizations or societies, and acceptable case law precedents make up the:
a. patient's right to emergency care
b. standard of care
c. local tort laws
d. civil EMS code

8. Generally, if there are no written Do Not Resuscitate (DNR) orders:
a. attempt to contact the family doctor before starting CPR
b. begin resuscitation efforts
c. consult law enforcement officers on the legality of starting CPR
d. accept the family's word that DNR orders exist

9. To refuse medical care, the patient must:
a. refuse any and all care the EMT may provide
b. be 15 years of age or older
c. not have received any medical care prior to the point of refusing
d. be mentally competent

10. An EMT may be required to report a suspected situation involving:
a. abuse of a child
b. commission of a crime
c. abuse of the elderly
d. all of the above

AMBULANCE OPERATIONS

11. The most important safety equipment in an ambulance:
a. are goggles and hard hats
b. are safety belts
c. is a fire extinguisher
d. are traffic flares

12. Most accidents involving emergency vehicles occur:
a. due to skids
b. during U-turns
c. en route to the hospital
d. at intersections

13. The recommended number of feet an ambulance should be parked from wreckage is:
a. 50
b. 100
c. 150
d. 200

14. Ambulances should be escorted by police or other emergency vehicles:
a. only if the crew is unfamiliar with the location of the patient or receiving facility
b. whenever possible
c. whenever responding to a potentially violent situation
d. only when the ambulance driver is inexperienced

15. A helicopter landing zone should ideally:
a. be a maximum of 90 feet by 90 feet square
b. be fenced off to keep onlookers away
c. be 100 feet by 100 feet square
d. have no more than a 15-degree slope

16. A medical helicopter should be approached:
a. from the rear
b. immediately after it lands
c. from the front
d. in a standing position

17. The "2-second rule" refers to:
a. the amount of time the ambulance should remain stopped at a traffic light before proceeding
b. the length of time a driver should look in the sideview mirror
c. the maximum amount of time it should take an EMT to make a driving decision
d. the distance that should be maintained between the ambulance and the vehicle in front of it

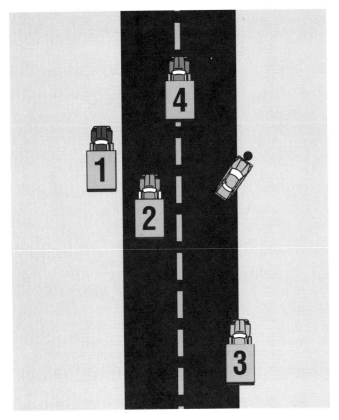

Figure 15-1

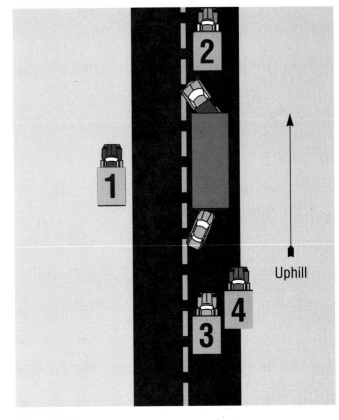

Figure 15-2

 18. Before crossing an intersection, the emergency vehicle driver should:
   a. look to the left, then to the right, and then again to the left
   b. turn off the siren and listen for other emergency vehicles
   c. look to the right, and then the left
   d. turn on the vehicle's 4-way flashers

19. Your unit responds to the scene of an auto accident where a vehicle has struck a tree. The road is a level 2-lane street with 2-way traffic. No police units are available to provide traffic control. Referring to Figure 15-1, the best place to position the ambulance would be location:
   a. 1
   b. 2
   c. 3
   d. 4

20. While travelling uphill, a car runs underneath the back end of a tanker truck carrying diesel fuel. There is no leakage present at this time, although the integrity of the tank is questionable. Referring to Figure 15-2, the best place to position the ambulance would be location:
   a. 1
   b. 2
   c. 3
   d. 4

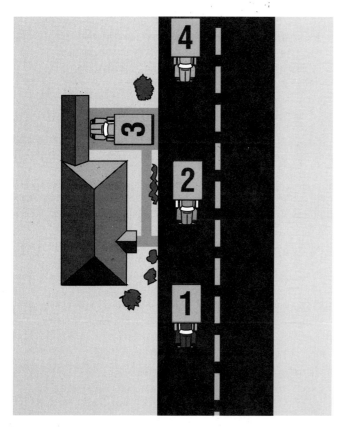

Figure 15-3

* **21.** You are dispatched to the scene of a domestic squabble that resulted in a shooting. As you near the house in a quiet suburban neighborhood, the communications center advises that police units are en route but will not arrive before your unit. Referring to Figure 15-3, the safest place to park your vehicle would be location:
   a. 1
   b. 2
   c. 3
   d. 4

PATIENT LIFTING AND MOVING

22. Lifting should be done using the:
   a. legs
   b. arms
   c. back
   d. waist

23. When lifting, keep the weight:
   a. as far from the body as possible
   b. a comfortable distance from the body
   c. as close to the body as possible
   d. to the right side of the body

24. Prior to lifting, the feet should be:
   a. together
   b. shoulder-width apart
   c. one in front of the other
   d. as far apart as possible

25. When lifting a stretcher or backboard, keep the back:
   a. locked into normal curvature
   b. bent forward
   c. bent backward
   d. twisted to one side

26. When grasping a stretcher, place the hands:
   a. next to each other
   b. at least 6 inches apart
   c. at least 10 inches apart
   d. at least 18 inches apart

27. If possible, lifting partners should:
   a. be approximately the same age
   b. have different amounts of physical strength
   c. be approximately the same height
   d. be of the same sex

28. Unless there is a medical contraindication, the best way to move a patient up or down stairs is with:
   a. a backboard
   b. a scoop stretcher
   c. an ambulance cot
   d. a stair chair

29. When reaching:
   a. do not reach more than 15–20 inches
   b. do not reach for more than 30 seconds
   c. try to reach to the side
   d. all of the above

30. Whenever possible in situations involving pulling or pushing:
   a. keep the elbows locked
   b. it is preferable to push rather than pull
   c. keep the weight below waist level
   d. keep the line of pull to the side of the body

31. The danger of moving a patient too soon is:
   a. further injury or illness may occur if the patient is not properly packaged
   b. a proper exam cannot be performed when a patient is on an ambulance cot
   c. the patient may wish to wait for the arrival of relatives before being transported
   d. there may not have been enough time to obtain consent to treat

32. An emergency move is used when:
   a. the patient's condition may deteriorate
   b. there are not enough EMTs to properly move the patient
   c. there is an immediate threat to the life of the patient
   d. maximum control of the spine is needed

33. If an emergency move must be made:
   a. roll the patient
   b. pull the patient in the direction of the long axis of the body
   c. pull the patient sideways in the direction of the shoulders
   d. lift the patient in any way possible and carry him or her

34. When performing an emergency move on a person injured in an auto accident:
   a. one EMT must continue to maintain cervical spinal immobilization
   b. take extra time to properly immobilize the spine
   c. there is no time to perform spinal immobilization
   d. a backboard is not used

35. The two types of nonemergency moves commonly used to move a patient from the ground to the stretcher when no injuries to the spine or extremities are suspected are the:
   a. power lift and leg lift
   b. direct ground lift and extremity lift
   c. immediate lift and nonemergency lift
   d. stretcher lift and backboard lift

36. The two primary methods used to transfer a patient from a bed to a stretcher are the:
   a. push method and pull method
   b. slide method and roll method
   c. immediate method and emergency method
   d. direct carry method and draw-sheet method

37. When using a wheeled stretcher:
   a. three EMTs are needed
   b. the EMTs should stand at the sides
   c. the foot end should be pulled
   d. smooth terrain should be avoided

38. When moving a wheeled stretcher over rough terrain, use:
   a. two rescuers, with one rescuer placed at each end facing each other
   b. two rescuers, with one rescuer placed at each end facing the same direction
   c. four rescuers, with one rescuer at each end facing each other and one rescuer on each side facing each other
   d. four rescuers, with one rescuer placed at each corner of the stretcher

39. When two patients on backboards are to be transported in the same ambulance, load the:
   a. patient who is to be placed on the ambulance benchseat first
   b. patient who will stay on the wheeled stretcher first
   c. heaviest patient first
   d. most critical patient first

40. A type of patient lifting device that can be separated lengthwise into halves and placed under a patient without log-rolling and with a minimum amount of movement is a:
a. basket stretcher
b. scoop stretcher
c. pole stretcher
d. SKED device

41. Using the following list of patient positions, mark the position most likely to be used to transport a patient suffering from the various problems listed:

legs elevated 8–12 inches; on left side; position of comfort; supine on backboard

_____ conscious patient who is nauseated or vomiting
_____ hypotensive pregnant patient
_____ patient complaining of severe difficulty breathing
_____ semiconscious seizure patient
_____ patient with chest pain
_____ spinal injury patient
_____ patient with a medical or nontraumatic head injury
_____ patient displaying signs of shock without spinal injury

GAINING ACCESS

42. When arriving at the scene of a vehicle crash, the first thing an EMT should do is:
a. make sure the scene is safe
b. assess the patient's airway
c. gain access to the patient
d. stabilize the vehicle

43. As a general rule, when dealing with downed wires at a crash scene:
a. there is no danger if they are telephone wires
b. manipulation is possible using heavy gloves
c. there is no danger if they are cable television wires
d. always consider wires energized

44. If a downed power line is in contact with a car at the scene of a crash, the best course of action is to:
a. wait for the electric company
b. remove the wire with a hotstick
c. tell the occupants to jump clear of the car
d. remove the wire with lineman's gloves

45. The best way to gain access to a patient who is still in a vehicle following a crash is to:
a. pry open the door closest to the patient with a crowbar or hydraulic tool
b. break a side window farthest from the patient and crawl in
c. have the patient reach over and unlock an undamaged door
d. check all doors to see if one will open

46. During the extrication process, patient care is generally:
a. discontinued until the patient is out of the vehicle
b. limited to assessment and vital signs
c. continued to the greatest extent possible
d. performed by firefighters

47. During the extrication process, the patient should be:
a. protected by a heavy, fireproof covering, and a rescuer should remain in the vehicle
b. protected by a heavy, fireproof covering and be left alone in the vehicle
c. restrained
d. covered with wet blankets to reduce fire hazard

MULTIPLE-CASUALTY SITUATIONS

48. The responsibility of the EMS unit that arrives first at a mass casualty incident is to:
a. immediately transport the most critical patients to the nearest hospital
b. assume command, assess the situation, and not perform patient care
c. start extricating patients
d. start caring for the most critically injured victims

49. A yellow triage tag signifies:
a. a second-priority patient
b. a patient who is a minor
c. a dead patient
d. a lowest-priority patient

50. The position of triage officer should be assigned to:
a. the highest ranking EMS officer
b. the EMT with the most seniority
c. the most competent EMT
d. a nurse, if available

51. A green triage tag signifies a patient:
a. with moderate-priority injuries
b. with low-priority injuries
c. who is suffering psychologic problems due to the incident
d. who is ready to be transported

52. Match the following sector officers with their primary responsibilities:
extrication sector; transportation sector; treatment sector; triage sector; staging sector; supply sector
_____ sorts patients based on medical priority
_____ obtains and distributes resources, such as medical equipment and personnel
_____ ascertains capabilities of receiving hospitals and coordinates loading of ambulances
_____ rescues patients who are trapped at the scene
_____ organizes incoming ambulances and coordinates the movement of ambulances to the loading zone
_____ coordinates medical care for injured patients after they have been sorted and moved

53. Using the following descriptions to prioritize patients at a mass casualty scene, categorize them as:
first, second, third, or fourth
(*Note:* If you normally use the color system, mark the patients as: **red, yellow, green, or black.**)
_____ severe head injury, no pulse or breathing
_____ severe burns
_____ multiple bone or joint injuries
_____ minor soft-tissue injuries
_____ unconsciousness of unknown cause
_____ back injury without spinal damage
_____ a severe medical problem
_____ shock
_____ swollen extremity accompanied by minor pain
_____ multiple traumatic injuries accompanied by full cardiac arrest
_____ burns without airway problems
_____ active labor with a breech presentation

54. A red triage tag signifies a patient who is:
a. a highest-priority patient
b. bleeding
c. a delayed-transport patient
d. burned

WELL-BEING OF THE EMT

55. The three ways communicable diseases are normally transmitted include all of the following *except:*
a. direct contact
b. casual contact
c. inhalation
d. indirect contact

56. Patients with communicable diseases:
a. can be easily identified by experienced EMTs
b. generally look ill
c. do not have a particular appearance
d. pose no threat to an EMT wearing protective gear

57. As an advanced safety precaution, it is generally recommended that an EMT receive an immunization to guard against:
a. HIV
b. tuberculosis
c. AIDS
d. hepatitis B

58. Gloves worn to protect the EMT against exposure to body fluids are most commonly made of:
a. vinyl or latex
b. rubber or butyl
c. butyl or vinyl
d. latex or rubber

59. As a general rule concerning the use of gloves:
a. there are some situations in which gloves may not be needed
b. gloves must be worn whenever a patient is being touched
c. gloves are only needed if blood is present
d. the decision to wear gloves can be made based on the type of dispatch

60. Hand washing should be performed:
a. only if the EMT was not wearing gloves
b. for at least 10–15 seconds
c. at least twice during a shift
d. using only a bactericidal cleaner

61. EMTs should wear protective eyewear:
a. whenever a patient with an infectious disease is encountered
b. only if they are susceptible to eye infections
c. if they have been recently ill
d. in situations where blood splatter may occur

62. When a patient suspected of having tuberculosis is encountered, wear:
a. SCBA
b. a disposable surgical mask
c. appropriate respiratory protection
d. a full face shield

63. Gowns should be worn when the EMT:
a. is working with a patient with a communicable disease
b. expects to have direct contact with a patient
c. expects to encounter large amounts of blood or body fluids
d. does not have a commercially manufactured EMS uniform

64. The HIV virus can be transmitted in all of the following ways *except:*
a. sharing intravenous drug needles and syringes
b. sexual contact
c. casual contact
d. from an infected mother to her baby

65. A federal agency that develops and enforces many regulations regarding infection control guidelines that apply to EMTs is the:
a. Department of Transportation (DOT)
b. National Highway Traffic Safety Administration (NHTSA)
c. National Fire Protection Association (NFPA)
d. Occupational Safety and Health Administration (OSHA)

66. After transporting an infectious disease patient, clean the ambulance by:
a. washing with a germicidal and viricidal agent
b. airing it out
c. wiping all surfaces with alcohol
d. using a commercially available aerosol spray

67. If it is known in advance that a patient with an infectious disease is to be transported:
a. remove unnecessary equipment from the ambulance prior to responding to the call
b. refuse to respond to the call
c. attempt to convince the patient to be transported by a friend or family member
d. remove all linens from the ambulance cot and cover it with plastic sheets

68. One of the best ways to protect against infectious disease is to:
    a. wear a mask and gown on all runs
    b. wash your hands after every run
    c. screen patients and not transport those with infectious diseases
    d. ride in the cab when a patient with an infectious disease is being transported

69. If called to a scene where the death of a patient is imminent:
    a. immediately transport the patient to a hospital
    b. have the family leave the room
    c. allow the family to be with the patient
    d. leave the patient in the care of law enforcement officials

70. To help the body deal with stress, increase intake of:
    a. carbohydrates
    b. caffeine
    c. sugar
    d. fatty foods

71. The purpose of Critical Incident Stress Management (CISM) is to:
    a. allow EMTs to talk to a psychiatrist
    b. identify EMTs who require disciplinary action
    c. identify things that were done wrong during an emergency
    d. help EMTs work through their emotional and physical responses to an incident

72. Ideally, a CISM team should be contacted:
    a. no later than 24 hours after the incident
    b. within 24 to 72 hours after the incident
    c. 1 week from the incident
    d. within a month of the incident

73. An important professional attribute that the EMT should strive to demonstrate is:
    a. appearance
    b. gaining initial training
    c. taking care of the patient regardless of the circumstances
    d. all of the above

HAZARDOUS MATERIALS

74. The primary responsibility of an EMT at an incident involving hazardous materials is:
    a. identifying the hazardous material
    b. controlling any spills or leaks
    c. the safety of himself or herself, the public, and the patients
    d. removing patients from the immediate vicinity of the hazardous material

75. Hazardous materials transported by motor vehicles may be identified by:
    a. calling the DOT
    b. obtaining a sample and sending it to a laboratory
    c. referencing the number on the placard
    d. smelling or feeling the substance

76. Information about a hazardous material used at an industrial or commercial site is best obtained:
    a. from the NFPA 704 symbol on the building
    b. from a material safety data sheet
    c. by interviewing plant employees
    d. by reading the label of the container from which the substance came

77. Generally, an EMT should enter an area where hazardous materials are found:
    a. anytime a patient's life is in danger
    b. if the EMT has completed a HAZMAT awareness course
    c. whenever firefighting turnout gear is available
    d. only if the EMT has proper training and is wearing HAZMAT equipment and SCBA

78. EMS vehicles and personnel at a scene involving hazardous materials should be positioned:
    a. close enough to quickly reach anyone who is sick or injured as a result of the incident
    b. upwind from the incident, and at safe distance
    c. downwind from the incident
    d. within shouting distance in the event that assistance is needed

ADDITIONAL POINTS FOR DISCUSSION

1. What office in your state certifies and governs EMTs? What is the address and phone number?

2. Does your state recognize DNR orders? Is there a standard state form? Does it have to be signed by the patient's doctor? What are your local and departmental procedures for dealing with a DNR order?

3. Review your department's guidelines for performing a mechanical check on the ambulance and for performing an inventory check of supplies.

4. What criteria does your department follow for deciding when to call for helicopter transport?

5. What are the guidelines of the local helicopter service for establishing a landing zone?

6. What are your state laws regarding:

   * Motorists yielding the right-of-way to emergency vehicles?

   * Driving emergency vehicles?

   * The use of red lights and sirens?

   * Operating an ambulance through a school zone and passing a school bus while on an emergency run?

7. If the ambulance is involved in an accident:

   * Which police units would be responsible for investigating the incident and filing a report?

   * Is there a specific form (departmental, county, or state) that must be completed?

8. What are some common situations (such as where there is a potential for violence directed at EMTs or potential situations involving hazardous materials) that may be encountered in your area that could be potentially dangerous for EMS personnel?

   What might you be able to do to protect yourself or minimize the chances of becoming involved in such a situation?

9. What is the role of your EMS crew at the scene of a vehicle crash involving entrapment?

10. What is the role of your EMS crew at an incident involving hazardous materials?

11. Is there a hazardous materials team available in your area? When would you summon this team and how?

12. What hazardous materials reference books are carried on the ambulance? Where are they kept?

13. Review your department's guidelines for:

   * Dealing with patients with infectious diseases

   * Reporting exposure to an infectious disease

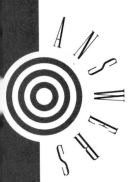

15 MISCELLANEOUS

1. **d.** Duty to act refers to the responsibility of an EMT, either by statute or function, to provide patient care when the opportunity presents itself.

2. **c.** Deviating from the accepted standard of care that a reasonable, prudent EMT would render is considered negligence.

3. **c.** Implied consent allows the EMT to assist an unconscious patient or a child if a true emergency situation exists. The basis of implied consent is that a rational and reasonable person who is similarly ill or injured but able to communicate would want medical care.

4. **d.** Abandonment is terminating care of a patient without assuring continuation of care at the same level or higher, or without the patient's consent to stop rendering care.

5. **a.** The four components necessary to prove negligence are a duty to act, breach of duty, an injury, and proximate cause.

6. **a.** Because they are important safeguards in protecting EMTs, EMS reports and records must be thorough and accurate. No one has a memory good enough to remember everything about a call, and lawsuits may occur years later. The EMS report is a legal document that is admissible in court. The document, if sloppy and incomplete, can be detrimental as it implies that the EMT's abilities are also sloppy and incomplete. Testimony from memory may not be enough—the court will generally view a procedure or action that is not documented as not having been performed.

7. **b.** The standard of care is established by local and state laws or protocols, professional organizations or societies, and acceptable case law precedents.

8. **b.** Although EMTs should honor written DNR orders, it is generally recommended that resuscitation efforts be started if the DNR orders are not present.

9. d. To refuse medical care, the patient must be mentally competent. A patient is allowed to refuse a particular form of therapy or one aspect of care. The patient can refuse further care after the EMT has started treatment procedures. Although there are some exceptions, patients generally must be at least 18 years of age to refuse treatment.

10. d. In most areas, EMTs are required to report a situation that they suspect involves abuse of a child or the elderly, or the commission of a crime.

11. b. Safety belts are the most important safety equipment in an ambulance and should be used by all personnel.

12. d. Approximately 50% of accidents involving emergency vehicles occur at intersections. 25% of emergency vehicle accidents occur while the vehicle is in reverse.

13. b. It is generally recommended that an ambulance be parked at least 100 feet from wreckage.

14. a. If the crew is unfamiliar with how to get to the location of the patient or how to get to the receiving facility, it is generally acceptable for the police or other emergency vehicles to escort an ambulance. Even in these cases, however, escorts should be avoided if possible because of the dangers involved in escort situations. In these cases, it is best if an experienced driver is operating the ambulance.

15. c. Ideally, a helicopter landing zone should be at least 100 feet by 100 feet square. The ground should have no more than a 10 degree slope and should be clear of fences or other obstructions.

16. c. Most medical helicopters should only be approached from the front, and approach only after being directed to do so by the pilot or flight crew. Stay low when approaching the helicopter, as rotor blades can dip low to the ground and cause injury.

17. d. The "2-second rule" refers to the distance that should be maintained between an emergency vehicle and the vehicle in front of it. Using a fixed object as a reference point, it should take the emergency vehicle at least 2 seconds to reach the object after the vehicle ahead has passed the object. This following distance should be increased if driving conditions are hazardous or if the emergency vehicle is a large fire or rescue truck.

18. a. Before crossing an intersection, the emergency vehicle driver should look to the left, then to the right, and then again to the left.

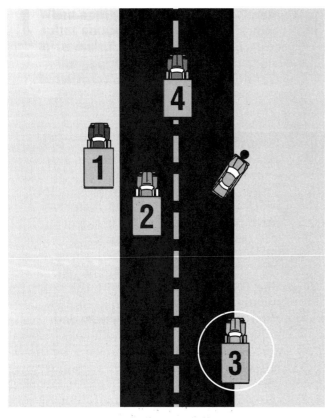

Figure 15-1

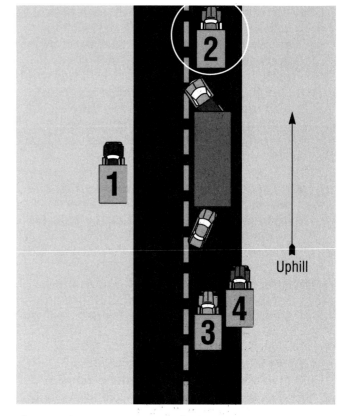

Uphill

Figure 15-2

19. **c.** Because police units will not be available to provide traffic control, location 3 would be the best place to position the ambulance. This provides protection for the patient in the car as well as the EMTs while only causing minimal traffic obstruction. The ambulance should not be placed where it is a hazard to oncoming traffic (as in locations 2 and 4), nor should it be placed where the safety of personnel could be jeopardized by having to cross the road (location 1). If police units are available to block traffic, the ambulance can be pulled beyond the accident and to the right side of the road.

20. **b.** Due to the nature of the accident, location 2 would be the best location to position the ambulance. It is uphill, and does not block traffic. Although a leak is not present, locations 3 and 4 are potentially dangerous if a leak develops because they are downhill. Additionally, if either accident vehicle is not stabilized, a danger of rolling is present. Location 1, although uphill, would place personnel in danger while trying to cross traffic.

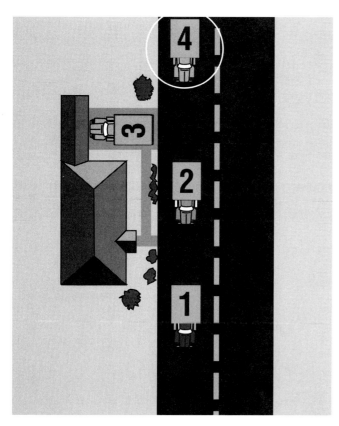

Figure 15-3

21. **d.** Domestic violence situations can be hazardous to EMTs, and positioning the unit is important. Location 4 allows the EMTs to view the house for possible hazards while being in a position to back out of the scene quickly if the perpetrator appears with a weapon. Once the police arrive, the crew can quickly access the patient when the scene is made secure. Location 1 would require the unit to drive past the front of the house, thereby placing the crew in the line of fire. Locations 2 and 3 obviously place the crew in great danger, as there is a direct line of fire available to the gunman. Location 3 also necessitates backing up in order to escape the scene.

22. **a.** Lifting should be done using the legs, not the back.

23. **c.** Keep the weight as close to the body as possible during lifting.

24. **b.** Keep the feet shoulder-width apart to provide firm footing during lifting.

25. **a.** Keep the back locked into normal curvature when lifting a stretcher or backboard.

26. **c.** Place the hands at least 10 inches apart when grasping a stretcher.

27. **c.** Ideally, lifting partners should be approximately the same height and strength. It is not necessary for them to be the same sex or of similar ages.

28. **d.** Unless there is a medical contraindication, a stair chair is ideal for moving a patient up or down stairs.

29. **a.** When reaching, do not reach distances more than 15–20 inches. Avoid twisting when reaching, and do not reach for periods longer than 1 minute.

30. **b.** Whenever possible, the EMT should push rather than pull.

31. **a.** The danger of moving a patient too soon is that further injury or illness may occur if the patient is not properly packaged. A full exam can be performed after the patient has been moved to the cot. Do not delay transport to wait for relatives or friends.

32. **c.** An emergency move is used when there is an immediate threat to the life of the patient. It is also used when lifesaving care cannot be rendered due to the patient's location or position, such as when a cardiac arrest patient is found sitting in a chair.

33. **b.** If an emergency move must be made, pull the patient in the direction of the long axis of the body, if possible.

34. a. When performing an emergency move on a person injured in an auto accident, there is not enough time to apply a short backboard or vest-style extrication device. However, one EMT must continue to manually maintain spinal immobilization. A cervical collar should be applied, if doing so will not add an inordinate amount of time to the extrication. When moving the patient to the backboard, cervical spine control can be provided manually.

35. b. If there is no suspected injury to the spine or extremities, the direct ground lift and extremity lift are two types of nonemergency moves that can be used to move a patient from the ground to a stretcher.

36. d. The direct carry and the draw-sheet method are two methods used to transfer a patient from a bed to a stretcher.

37. c. When using a wheeled stretcher, the foot end should be pulled. Two EMTs can use a wheeled stretcher and should be positioned at each end. This device works best over smooth terrain.

38. d. When a wheeled stretcher must be moved over rough terrain, use four rescuers with one placed at each corner of the stretcher.

39. a. When two patients on backboards are to be transported in one ambulance, the patient who is to be placed on the ambulance benchseat should be loaded first. Do not attempt to move a patient on a backboard over another patient on the ambulance stretcher.

40. b. The scoop stretcher can be separated lengthwise into halves and slid under the patient with a minimal amount of movement. This type of stretcher is ideal for moving a patient up or down steps once the patient is secured with straps.

41.

position of comfort	conscious patient who is nauseated or vomiting
on left side	hypotensive pregnant patient
position of comfort	patient complaining of severe difficulty breathing
on left side	semiconscious seizure patient
position of comfort	patient with chest pain
supine on backboard	spinal injury patient
on left side	patient with a medical or nontraumatic head injury
legs elevated 8–12″	patient displaying signs of shock without spinal injury

42. a. The first thing the EMT should do when arriving at the scene of an auto accident is to make sure the scene is safe. This includes checking for downed wires, fire hazards, and other dangers. The safety of the EMTs and rescuers must come first.

43. d. Always consider any downed wire energized and dangerous. Even a cable television or telephone wire may be energized if it has come in contact with electric wires down-line. Never attempt to manipulate the wire unless local protocols and proper training dictate otherwise.

44. a. The best course of action when energized wires have contacted a car is to wait for the electric company. Occupants should only be instructed to jump clear of the car if they are in immediate danger from fire or another life-threatening situation.

45. d. To gain access to a patient, check all the doors first. Although the EMT may be unable to open the door closest to the patient, other doors may be usable. Remember to "Try before you pry." If the doors will not open, it may be possible to roll down a window for access. Although the patient may be able to unlock a door, this may not be desirable if it will further aggravate an injury.

46. c. Generally, necessary care should be continued to the greatest extent possible during the extrication process.

47. a. During the extrication process, patients should be properly protected by a heavy, fireproof covering. A rescuer should also remain in the vehicle to monitor the patient and provide reassurance.

48. b. The first EMS unit to arrive at a mass casualty scene should assume medical command, assess the situation, start calling for additional aid, and direct incoming units. Patient care should not be started by this unit. Clear command must be established early if the incident is to be managed in an orderly fashion. If enough EMTs are present, triage may also be started.

49. a. A yellow triage tag signifies a second-priority or moderately injured patient.

50. c. The most competent EMT should assume the role of triage officer. Rank and seniority are unimportant at the scene of a mass casualty. Nurses, unless specially trained, lack the experience and expertise necessary to properly triage patients in the field.

51. b. A green triage tag signifies a patient with minor injuries. These are delayed-priority patients. Patients with green tags are sometimes referred to as the "walking wounded." This is not an appropriate term, however, because some walking patients may have severe injuries, and some patients with minor injuries may not be able to walk.

52.

triage sector	sorts patients based on medical priority
supply sector	obtains and distributes resources, such as medical equipment and personnel
transportation sector	ascertains capabilities of receiving hospitals and coordinates loading of ambulances
extrication sector	rescues patients who are trapped at the scene
staging sector	organizes incoming ambulances and coordinates the movement of ambulances to the loading zone
treatment sector	coordinates medical care for injured patients after they have been sorted and moved

53.

__fourth (black)__	severe head injury, no pulse or breathing
__first (red)__	severe burns
__second (yellow)__	multiple bone or joint injuries
__third (green)__	minor soft-tissue injuries
__first (red)__	unconsciousness of unknown cause
__second (yellow)__	back injury without spinal damage
__first (red)__	a severe medical problem
__first (red)__	shock
__third (green)__	swollen extremity accompanied by minor pain
__fourth (black)__	multiple traumatic injuries accompanied by full cardiac arrest
__second (yellow)__	burns without airway problems
__first (red)__	active labor with a breech presentation

54. **a.** A red triage tag signifies a critical, first-priority patient.

55. **b.** Communicable diseases are normally transmitted by direct contact, indirect contact, or inhalation. They are not normally transmitted by casual contact.

56. **c.** An EMT cannot recognize a patient with a communicable disease simply by his or her appearance.

57. **d.** Because EMS personnel are at greatest risk from hepatitis B, it is generally recommended that an EMT receive a hepatitis B immunization.

58. **a.** Gloves worn by EMTs are most commonly made from vinyl or latex. They may also be made of nitrile.

59. **a.** Gloves protect from diseases transmitted by a variety of other body fluids aside from blood, and local protocols regarding their use should always be followed. There are some situations where gloves may not be needed, however, such as when caring for a patient with a closed injury to the wrist or ankle.

60. **b.** When washing the hands, wash for at least 10–15 seconds. Hands should be washed after patient contact and after using the restroom. Hands should still be washed even if gloves were worn. Although antimicrobial or bactericidal cleaners are ideal, simple soap and water provides adequate protection against germs and bacteria.

61. **d.** In situations where blood may splatter, wear protective eyewear.

62. **c.** Wear appropriate respiratory protection, such as a HEPA (High Efficiency Particulate Air) respirator when working around a patient suspected of having tuberculosis. Always follow local protocols.

63. **c.** When the EMT expects to encounter large amounts of blood or body fluid, it is advisable to put on a gown if time permits.

64. **c.** HIV is primarily transmitted by the sharing of intravenous drug needles and syringes, by sexual contact, and from an infected mother to her baby. It is also transmitted by blood transfusions. Casual contact has not been linked to HIV transmission.

65. **d.** The Occupational Safety and Health Administration (OSHA) develops and enforces many regulations regarding infection control guidelines for health care workers. EMS is subject to these regulations.

66. **a.** After transporting a patient with a communicable disease, the inside of the ambulance should be washed with a germicidal and viricidal agent. The use of aerosol sprays is not recommended, as very little of the agent may reach the surface to be cleaned. Instead, use trigger-pump spray bottles to deliver the agent. Alcohol does not kill the germs and viruses. Research has shown that airing out an ambulance is of no benefit.

67. **a.** If it is known in advance that a patient with an infectious disease is to be transported, unnecessary equipment may be removed from the ambulance to prevent contamination. A truly sick patient should be transported by ambulance. Linens may be exchanged or discarded at the hospital, but should not be replaced with uncomfortable plastic sheets simply to avoid using linens.

68. **b.** Thoroughly wash the hands preferably with a germicidal and viricidal solution, following each run. Additional protection can be gained by having yearly physical checkups and current vaccinations. It is not always necessary to wear a mask and gown, nor should the patient be left alone in the back of the ambulance.

69. **c.** If death is imminent, the family should be allowed to be with the patient whenever possible. It may not be appropriate to transport the patient to the hospital, for example, if there is a written DNR order on hand.

70. **a.** To help the body deal with stress, increase intake of carbohydrates. Decrease intake of caffeine, alcohol, sugar, and fat.

71. **d.** The purpose of Critical Incident Stress Management (CISM) is to help EMTs work through their emotional and physical responses to an incident and to accelerate the recovery process. It is not a disciplinary procedure designed to discuss mistakes or areas that need improvement.

72. **b.** Ideally, a CISM team should be contacted within 24 to 72 hours after the critical incident.

73. **a.** There are a number of important professional attributes an EMT should strive to demonstrate, including a neat, presentable appearance. Initial training is just a start, and continuing education is necessary to keep knowledge and skills up-to-date. Remember, it is not whether you are paid or not that makes you a professional. Your attitude makes you a professional.

74. **c.** The primary responsibility of an EMT at an incident involving hazardous materials is the safety of himself or herself, the public, and the patients. Access to patients should be accomplished only after personnel are properly protected with appropriate gear and breathing apparatus. Although early identification of the substance is important, it does not take priority over safety considerations. Identification of the substance is usually the responsibility of the fire department or hazardous materials team. Controlling the actual incident is not usually the job of EMS personnel.

75. **c.** Identification of hazardous materials transported by motor vehicles is best made by referencing the four-digit guide number on the placard and shipping information. The vehicle operator may not know what is being carried, and laboratory testing is a time-consuming process. Never smell or touch a potentially hazardous material. Identification should always be made while the EMT remains at a safe distance from the incident.

76. **b.** Information about a hazardous material used at an industrial or commercial site is best obtained by referencing a material safety data sheet. Plant employees may not be familiar with the material or may provide inaccurate information, and the container may be misleading.

77. **d.** Generally, only EMTs with proper training in wearing HAZMAT equipment and SCBA should enter an area where hazardous materials are found.

78. **b.** EMS vehicles and personnel at a scene involving hazardous materials should be positioned upwind from the incident and at a safe distance. Shouting distance is normally much too close, as fumes may quickly reach EMS personnel. In most instances, patients should be brought to the EMT, unless the EMT is properly trained and protected to enter the scene.

CPR/BLS AND AIRWAY OBSTRUCTION

1. It is important for an EMT to have a good working knowledge of BLS because:
   a. most patients transported by ambulance need CPR
   b. most people having cardiac emergencies arrest before reaching the hospital
   c. EMTs very often become CPR instructors
   d. a large percentage of cardiac arrests occur outside of the hospital

2. The percentage of oxygen present in room air is:
   a. 21
   b. 35
   c. 56
   d. 78

3. The percentage of oxygen in exhaled air is approximately:
   a. 5
   b. 16
   c. 21
   d. 78

4. Early opening of the airway and performance of artificial ventilation is important because brain damage can occur within:
   a. 2–4 minutes
   b. 4–6 minutes
   c. 8–10 minutes
   d. 10–12 minutes

5. In an unconscious patient, the most common cause of airway obstruction is:
   a. the tongue
   b. food
   c. blood
   d. small toys or marbles

6. After assuring scene safety and taking body substance isolation precautions, the first thing a rescuer should do when a patient has collapsed due to illness or injury is:
   a. open the airway
   b. check for a medic-alert tag
   c. call for help
   d. determine whether the patient is unresponsive

7. The preferred method of opening the airway of a patient without suspected spinal injury is the:
   a. head tilt/neck lift
   b. modified jaw thrust
   c. Heimlich maneuver
   d. head tilt/chin lift

8. The preferred method of opening the airway of a patient with a suspected neck injury is the:
   a. head tilt/chin lift
   b. head tilt/neck lift
   c. modified jaw thrust
   d. Heimlich maneuver

9. After opening the airway, check for breathing for:
   a. 1–3 seconds
   b. 3–5 seconds
   c. 5–10 seconds
   d. at least 10 seconds

10. If an adult patient is not breathing, deliver:
    a. four quick breaths
    b. two slow breaths if alone, four quick breaths if a partner is present
    c. two full breaths 1½ to 2 seconds in duration
    d. one full breath 1 to 1½ seconds in duration

11. Ventilate an adult patient who is not breathing but has a pulse at a rate of:
    a. 6–10 times a minute, once every 6–10 seconds
    b. 10–12 times a minute, once every 5–6 seconds
    c. 12–15 times a minute, once every 4–5 seconds
    d. 15–20 times a minute, once every 3–4 seconds

12. For a laryngectomy patient, ventilations should be delivered through the patient's:
    a. mouth and nose
    b. stoma
    c. mouth
    d. nose

13. To locate the carotid pulse:
    a. place the thumb on one side of the trachea and the forefinger on the opposite side at the level of the Adam's apple
    b. place two fingers in the notch directly below the Adam's apple
    c. place the thumb on the Adam's apple, then slide it into the groove between the neck muscles and trachea
    d. place two fingers on the Adam's apple, then slide them into the groove between the neck muscles and trachea

14. Initially assess the pulse for:
    a. 5–10 seconds
    b. 10–15 seconds
    c. 30–45 seconds
    d. 60 seconds

15. To properly receive CPR, the patient must be:
    a. in the Trendelenburg position
    b. on a firm, flat surface
    c. at least 6 months of age
    d. in a prone position

16. To perform external chest compressions on an adult, use:
    a. two hands on a man, one hand on a woman
    b. the heel of one hand
    c. two hands, one placed on top of the other
    d. two hands, placed side by side

17. Chest compressions should be delivered to:
    a. the upper third of the sternum
    b. the xiphoid process
    c. the lower third of the sternum
    d. the manubrium

18. When adult CPR is being performed, the proper depth of chest compressions is:
    a. ¾–1½ inches
    b. 1½–2 inches
    c. 2–2½ inches
    d. as deep as necessary to produce a palpable pulse

19. Chest compressions should be:
  a. 25% compression, 75% relaxation
  b. 50% compression, 50% relaxation
  c. 75% compression, 25% percent relaxation
  d. varied for optimum output

20. The ratio of chest compressions to ventilations in one-rescuer adult CPR is:
  a. 5:2
  b. 15:1
  c. 5:1
  d. 15:2

21. On a per-minute basis in one-rescuer adult CPR, compressions should be delivered at a rate of:
  a. 60–80
  b. 80–100
  c. at least 60
  d. at least 100

22. When performing two-rescuer adult CPR:
  a. pause after the fifth compression to allow the second rescuer to deliver a breath
  b. deliver a breath on the downstroke of the fifth compression
  c. pause after the fifth compression to allow the second rescuer to deliver two full breaths
  d. the second rescuer delivers a breath whenever possible

23. Patients in cardiac arrest should be reassessed:
  a. every 5 minutes
  b. after the first minute of CPR and every 10 minutes thereafter
  c. after the first minute of CPR and every few minutes thereafter
  d. only if the patient starts breathing on his or her own

24. When resuming one-rescuer adult CPR after reassessing the patient, give:
  a. no breaths and resume compressions
  b. one breath and resume compressions
  c. two breaths and resume compressions
  d. two breaths and recheck the pulse

25. For adults, activate the EMS system after:
  a. checking for a pulse
  b. the patient resumes a spontaneous pulse and is breathing
  c. becoming too tired to continue CPR
  d. determining that the patient is unresponsive

26. To find the proper hand position for adult external chest compressions:
  a. measure two fingers below the middle of the sternum
  b. measure one finger above the xiphoid process
  c. measure two fingers above the manubrium
  d. measure one finger below the nipple line

27. The ratio of chest compressions to ventilations for two-rescuer adult CPR is:
  a. 5:1
  b. 15:2
  c. 5:2
  d. 15:1

28. For two-rescuer adult CPR, the rate of compressions on a per–minute basis is:
  a. at least 60
  b. 40–60
  c. 60–80
  d. 80–100

29. After reassessing the patient for return of breathing and circulation during two-rescuer adult CPR, the rescuer at the chest should:
  a. resume compressions after the rescuer at the head gives a breath
  b. pause after every four cycles of compressions to allow for a pulse check
  c. resume compressions without the rescuer at the head giving a breath
  d. intersperse an abdominal thrust after every cycle of five compressions

30. During two-rescuer CPR, a call for switching positions is made by the:
  a. rescuer performing ventilations
  b. rescuer performing compressions
  c. senior EMT
  d. rescuer who has been doing CPR the longest

31. After switching positions, the rescuer at the head:
   a. checks for a pulse and breathing
   b. immediately gives a breath
   c. waits for the rescuer at the chest to resume compressions
   d. gives two breaths and checks a pulse

32. Signs of effective CPR include all the following *except:*
   a. return of spontaneous pulses and breathing
   b. return of color to the patient (i.e., the patient "pinks" up)
   c. strong pulses with compressions
   d. dilated pupils

33. When performing CPR, use supplemental oxygen:
   a. after the first pulse check
   b. when the rescuer starts to tire of rescue breathing
   c. as soon as it is available
   d. only if there is no history of breathing problems

34. When managing a drowning patient in cardiac arrest:
   a. start chest compressions while the patient is still in the water
   b. wait until the patient is removed from the water to start CPR
   c. allow paramedics to assess the patient's EKG before starting CPR
   d. start ventilations while the patient is still in the water

35. If air does not seem to enter the lungs during attempts to ventilate an unconscious patient:
   a. reposition the head and neck and reattempt ventilation
   b. perform abdominal thrusts
   c. perform a finger sweep
   d. perform chest thrusts

36. When a conscious adult patient has an obstructed airway:
   a. perform six to ten abdominal thrusts
   b. administer four back blows followed by four abdominal thrusts
   c. perform abdominal thrusts until the obstruction is cleared or the patient becomes unconscious
   d. administer back blows only

37. A patient with a partial airway obstruction but good exchange of air should be:
   a. managed in the same way as a patient with a full obstruction
   b. encouraged to cough and monitored closely
   c. given back blows only
   d. encouraged to drink a large glass of water to dislodge the obstruction

38. To relieve an airway obstruction in a pregnant or obese patient, use:
   a. abdominal thrusts
   b. chest thrusts
   c. back blows
   d. the Heimlich maneuver

39. To manage an airway obstruction in an unconscious adult patient, repeat cycles of:
   a. four abdominal thrusts followed by four chest thrusts, then reattempt to ventilate
   b. five abdominal thrusts followed by a finger sweep, then attempt to ventilate
   c. five back blows followed by five abdominal thrusts, then attempt to ventilate
   d. six to ten abdominal thrusts followed by one ventilation, then a finger sweep

40. After a foreign body is successfully dislodged, the patient should be:
   a. told to rest and not to eat hard foods for a day or two
   b. advised to see their family physician the next day
   c. encouraged to go to a hospital and be examined by a physician
   d. observed for 5 minutes and sent home if no difficulties are noted

41. By American Heart Association (AHA) definition, a child is:
    a. 1–8 years old
    b. younger than 1 year old
    c. 2–10 years old
    d. 5–14 years old

42. To perform chest compressions on a child, use:
    a. the heel of one hand placed on the lower third of the sternum
    b. two hands placed on the middle of the sternum
    c. three fingers below the nipple line
    d. the heel of one hand placed on the upper half of the sternum

43. When chest compressions on a child are being done, the hand closest to the patient's forehead should be:
    a. placed over the hand that is on the sternum
    b. kept on the patient's forehead to maintain head tilt
    c. placed under the patient's neck to maintain head tilt
    d. used to continually monitor a carotid pulse

44. The chest of a child should be compressed:
    a. $\frac{1}{6}$ to $\frac{1}{4}$ the total depth of the chest
    b. $\frac{1}{4}$ to $\frac{1}{3}$ the total depth of the chest
    c. $\frac{1}{3}$ to $\frac{1}{2}$ the total depth of the chest
    d. $\frac{1}{2}$ to $\frac{2}{3}$ the total depth of the chest

45. If a child is not breathing but has a pulse, the patient should be be ventilated at a rate of:
    a. 10 times a minute, once every 6 seconds
    b. 12 times a minute, once every 5 seconds
    c. 15 times a minute, once every 4 seconds
    d. 20 times a minute, once every 3 seconds

46. By AHA definition, an infant is:
    a. younger than 1 year
    b. younger than 18 months old
    c. 1–2 years old
    d. newborn to 3 years old

47. To assess the pulse of an infant, check the:
    a. brachial pulse
    b. apical pulse
    c. carotid pulse
    d. radial pulse

48. When opening the airway of an infant, avoid:
    a. using the jaw-thrust method
    b. hyperextending the neck
    c. suctioning
    d. using the head-tilt/chin-lift method

49. When ventilating an infant:
    a. give full breaths
    b. administer rapid breaths $\frac{1}{2}$ to 1 second in duration
    c. perform mouth-to-mouth and nose breathing
    d. give four small puffs

50. To perform chest compression on an infant, use:
    a. two fingers placed on the upper sternum
    b. two fingers placed one finger width below the nipple line
    c. the heel of one hand placed on the middle of the sternum
    d. both thumbs placed on the upper sternum

51. The chest of an infant should be compressed:
    a. $\frac{1}{16}$ to $\frac{1}{8}$ the total depth of the chest
    b. $\frac{1}{8}$ to $\frac{1}{4}$ the total depth of the chest
    c. $\frac{1}{4}$ to $\frac{1}{3}$ the total depth of the chest
    d. $\frac{1}{3}$ to $\frac{1}{2}$ the total depth of the chest

52. For CPR on infants or children, the ratio of compressions to ventilations is:
    a. 15:2 regardless of the number of rescuers
    b. 5:1 for infants and 15:2 for children
    c. 15:2 for one-rescuer CPR
    d. 5:1 regardless of the number of rescuers

53. If an infant is not breathing but has a pulse, the patient should be be ventilated at a rate of:
a. 10 times a minute, once every 6 seconds
b. 12 times a minute, once every 5 seconds
c. 15 times a minute, once every 4 seconds
d. 20 times a minute, once every 3 seconds

54. A conscious infant with a complete airway obstruction may be identified by:
a. pink lips
b. an absent pulse
c. an inability to cry
d. a persistent, forceful cough

55. One difference between managing an infant with an airway obstruction as opposed to an adult is that:
a. back blows are not used
b. abdominal thrusts are interspersed with chest thrusts
c. ventilation is not attempted until the obstruction is relieved
d. chest thrusts are used instead of abdominal thrusts

56. To relieve an airway obstruction in an infant, perform cycles of:
a. six to ten abdominal thrusts
b. five back blows followed by five chest thrusts
c. six to ten chest thrusts followed by a finger sweep
d. five back blows followed by five abdominal thrusts

57. Manual removal of foreign bodies obstructing the airway in infants and children should be performed:
a. only on patients older than 5 years of age
b. only if the object can be visualized
c. by using a blind finger sweep
d. only on infants

58. When attempting to relieve an obstructed airway in an infant, position the infant:
a. with the head and shoulders elevated
b. with the head and trunk level
c. upside-down by the feet and ankles
d. with the head lower than the trunk

59. If a rescuer is alone and finds a child or infant without a pulse and who is not breathing:
a. perform CPR for 1 minute, then phone for help
b. immediately phone for help
c. perform CPR for 5 minutes, then phone for help
d. open the airway, give two slow breaths, then phone for help

60. CPR should not be interrupted:
a. when performing automated external defibrillation
b. for more than a few seconds except in special situations
c. for any reason
d. for more than a few minutes unless performing endotracheal intubation

61. CPR may be discontinued for any of the following reasons *except:*
a. the rescuer becomes too exhausted to continue
b. spontaneous ventilation and circulation are restored
c. the patient's pupils become fixed and dilated
d. an authorized individual pronounces the patient dead

62. All of the following statements concerning complications from CPR are true *except:*
a. they occur only when CPR is performed by poorly trained rescuers
b. they include injuries to the lungs, heart, liver, and spleen
c. they may occur even when compressions are properly performed
d. they include fractures of the ribs and sternum

63. When ventilating a person wearing dentures:
a. remove the dentures
b. remove the dentures only if it is a partial plate
c. leave the dentures in place
d. leave the dentures in place only if it is a partial plate

64. If slight gastric distention is noted during CPR:
   a. relieve the distention by exerting moderate pressure with one hand over the upper abdomen
   b. discontinue CPR
   c. reposition the airway and breathe less forcefully
   d. place the patient's head and neck in a neutral position

65. The chance of gastric distention and regurgitation can be reduced by:
   a. tilting the patient's head forward
   b. not using an adjunctive airway
   c. not pinching the patient's nose
   d. ventilating with less force and speed

ADDITIONAL POINTS FOR DISCUSSION

1. Identify specific buildings or locations in your area where it may be difficult to perform CPR while moving the patient.

   If the patient must be moved, how will this be accomplished?

ADDITIONAL BLS REVIEW

After completing the multiple-choice questions, fill in the appropriate answers in the chart below.
   1. Check for _____.
   2. Access the EMS system.
   3. Open _____ and check for _____.
   4. Give _____ if breathing is absent:
       _____ seconds each for adults.
       _____ seconds each for infants and children.
   5. Check for _____ and _____.

Summary of Adult One- and Two-Rescuer CPR

	One–Rescuer	Two–Rescuer
Rate:	_____	_____
Ratio:	_____	_____
Hand Placement:	_____	_____
Depth of Compressions:	_____	_____
Location of Pulse Check:	_____	_____
Rescue Breathing:	_____	_____

Summary of Infant and Child CPR

	Infant	Child
Age:	_____	_____
Rate:	_____	_____
Ratio:	_____	_____
Hand Placement:	_____	_____
Depth of Compressions:	_____	_____
Location of Pulse Check:	_____	_____
Rescue Breathing:	_____	_____

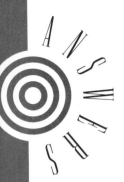

16 CPR/BLS

AND AIRWAY OBSTRUCTION

1. d. Because a large percentage of cardiac arrests occur outside of the hospital setting, it is imperative that EMTs have a good working knowledge of CPR and remain proficient in their skills. Not all patients experiencing cardiac emergencies will arrest, but the EMT must be ready if they do.

2. a. Oxygen makes up only 21% of room air.

3. b. Only 5% of the 21% of oxygen in room air is needed to sustain life. The air exhaled by a rescuer performing CPR contains 16% oxygen (21%–5%). This 16% oxygen exhaled by the rescuer is enough to sustain the life of the patient.

4. b. Without oxygen, brain damage occurs in 4–6 minutes.

5. a. The tongue is the most common cause of airway obstruction in an unconscious patient.

6. d. After assuring scene safety and taking body substance isolation precautions, the first step in Basic Life Support is to establish whether the patient is unresponsive. After establishing unresponsiveness, the rescuer should call for help and then open the airway.

7. d. The head-tilt/chin-lift maneuver is the preferred method of opening the airway of a patient without a suspected spinal injury. This method works better than the head tilt/neck lift because the chin lift moves the mandible forward, thereby lifting the tongue up and out of the oropharynx.

8. c. The modified jaw-thrust maneuver should be used to open the airway of a patient with a suspected neck injury.

9. b. Check for breathing for 3–5 seconds after opening the airway. To check, look for chest movement, listen for breathing, and feel with your cheek for air movement.

10. **c.** Two slow breaths of 1½ to 2 seconds in duration should be delivered to an adult patient who is not breathing. For infants and children, two slow breaths of 1 to 1½ seconds in duration should be delivered.

11. **b.** An adult patient who is not breathing but has a pulse should be ventilated at a rate of 10–12 times a minute, once every 5–6 seconds.

12. **b.** To ventilate a laryngectomy patient, ventilations should be delivered through the patient's stoma. To accomplish this, a child- or infant-sized ventilation mask can be placed over the stoma. Some patients may have only a partial or temporary tracheostomy. If this is the case, the rescuer may need to seal the patient's mouth and nose before ventilating to prevent air from leaking.

13. **d.** To locate the carotid pulse, place two fingers on the Adam's apple and slide them into the groove between the neck muscles and trachea toward the rescuer. Do not attempt to palpate the pulse on the side of the trachea opposite the rescuer, and do not use the thumb to check a pulse.

14. **a.** The patient's pulse should initially be assessed for 5–10 seconds.

15. **b.** The CPR patient must be on a firm, flat surface to properly receive CPR. The patient should be in a supine position (on his or her back). There are no age requirements to receive CPR.

16. **c.** External chest compressions on an adult are performed using two hands on the sternum. The heel of the rescuer's hand closest to the patient's head should be placed on the sternum, and the rescuer's other hand should be placed on top of it.

17. **c.** Chest compressions should be delivered to the lower third of the sternum. The manubrium is the upper portion of the sternum.

18. **b.** The depth for chest compressions performed on an adult patient is 1½ to 2 inches.

19. **b.** Compressions should be delivered in a smooth manner, with 50% compression and 50% relaxation. The hands should not be removed from the patient's chest during the relaxation period.

20. **d.** The correct ratio of compressions to ventilations in one-rescuer adult CPR is 15:2.

21. **b.** Compressions should be delivered at a rate of 80–100 per minute in one-rescuer adult CPR.

22. **a.** When performing two-rescuer adult CPR, the rescuer performing compressions should pause after the fifth compression to allow the second rescuer to ventilate the patient.

23. **c.** After the first minute of CPR, the patient's pulse and breathing should be reassessed. This equals four cycles of compressions and ventilations in one-rescuer adult CPR or 10 cycles in two-rescuer CPR. Thereafter, the patient should be reassessed every few minutes.

24. **a.** When resuming one-rescuer adult CPR after reassessing the patient, begin with chest compressions. Give no breaths prior to resuming compressions.

25. d. For adults, the EMS system should be activated immediately after determining that the patient is unresponsive. If the rescuer is alone, he or she should call for additional help. If someone else is available, that person should call while the rescuer continues assessing the patient. Early delivery of defibrillation and Advanced Life Support is critical to the survival of adult patients because ventricular fibrillation is the most common cause of arrest. If the rescuer is alone, rapid access to EMS may be more important than a short period of CPR, which will need to be interrupted anyway for help to be summoned.

26. b. Measure one finger above the xyphoid process to find the proper hand position for adult chest compressions. Using the hand closest to the patient's feet, place the middle finger over the xyphoid process and the index finger next to it. Then place the heel of the hand closest to the patient's head next to the index finger, thereby positioning the hand one finger above the xyphoid process.

27. a. The correct ratio of compressions to ventilations in two-rescuer adult CPR is 5:1.

28. d. In two-rescuer adult CPR, compressions should be delivered at a rate of 80–100 per minute, the same rate as for one-rescuer adult CPR.

29. c. When resuming two-rescuer adult CPR after reassessing the patient, the rescuer at the chest begins performing chest compressions. The rescuer at the head does not give a breath prior to resuming compressions. The pulse should be checked every few minutes thereafter.

30. b. The rescuer performing compressions initiates a change in positions. The call is usually made when the rescuer becomes fatigued.

31. a. After changing positions, the rescuer at the head checks for a pulse and breathing. If neither is present, he or she calls for resumption of CPR.

32. d. Dilated pupils are not a sign of effective CPR. Signs of effective CPR include a return of spontaneous pulses and breathing, return of color to the patient, and good pulses with compressions.

33. c. Supplemental oxygen should be used as soon as it becomes available during CPR. Any patient who is not breathing should be ventilated with 100% oxygen.

34. d. Ventilations should be started as soon as possible on drowning patients. If practical, this should be begun while the patient is still in the water. Because a hard surface is needed for chest compressions, patients normally have to be removed from the water before compressions are initiated. Compressions should not be initiated while patients are still in the water unless the rescuer has special training in performing in-water CPR.

35. a. The rescuer should reposition the airway and attempt to ventilate a second time if air does not seem to enter the patient's lungs initially.

36. c. If a conscious adult has a completely obstructed airway, the rescuer should perform abdominal thrusts until the obstruction is relieved or the patient becomes unconscious. Back blows are not used on adults.

37. b. A patient with a partial airway obstruction but good exchange of air should be encouraged to cough and monitored closely. A patient with a partial obstruction with poor air exchange should be managed in the same way as a patient with a complete obstruction.

38. **b.** Use chest thrusts instead of abdominal thrusts to relieve an airway obstruction in a pregnant or obese patient.

39. **b.** The rescuer should repeat cycles of up to five abdominal thrusts followed by a finger sweep and a ventilation attempt when managing an unconscious adult with an obstructed airway.

40. **c.** Patients who have experienced airway obstruction should be examined by a physician. Although the patient cannot be forced to go to a hospital, EMTs should strongly encourage the patient to do so. Trauma to the area of the larynx may not be readily recognized, and swelling may later compromise the airway.

41. **a.** By AHA standards, a child is a patient who is 1–8 years old.

42. **a.** The heel of one hand is used when performing CPR on a child. It is placed over the lower third of the sternum.

43. **b.** When compressions on a child are being done, the hand closest to the patient's head should be kept on the patient's forehead to maintain an open airway. After ventilating the patient, the rescuer replaces the hand performing compressions on the chest by sight.

44. **c.** The depth of compressions for CPR in children is approximately ⅓ to ½ the depth of the chest, which is about 1 to 1½ inches on most children.

45. **d.** To perform rescue breathing on a child who has a pulse but is not breathing, ventilate the patient 20 times a minute, once every 3 seconds. This is the same rate as for an infant.

46. **a.** By AHA standards, an infant is a patient younger than 1 year.

47. **a.** The brachial pulse is used to assess the pulse of an infant. The carotid pulse is used to assess the pulse of a child.

48. **b.** Avoid hyperextending the neck of an infant, which can be caused by excessive head tilt. The cartilaginous rings of the trachea are not fully formed; thus, hyperextension of the neck can kink the trachea (in the same way a garden hose may be kinked) and result in airway obstruction.

49. **c.** When ventilating an infant, the rescuer should cover the infant's mouth and nose with his or her mouth, or a mask. Ventilation should be slow puffs (1–1½ seconds in duration), to avoid high pressure and gastric distention.

50. **b.** Chest compressions should be performed by placing two fingers one finger width below an imaginary line drawn between the infant's nipples. For newborns, the rescuer may use two thumbs placed in the same location to perform compressions, and encircle the chest with the rest of the fingers.

51. **d.** The depth of compressions for infant CPR is approximately ⅓ to ½ the depth of the chest, which is about ½ to 1 inch on most infants.

52. **d.** The ratio of compressions to ventilations when performing CPR on infants or children is 5:1 regardless of the number of rescuers.

53. **d.** If an infant is not breathing but has a pulse, he or she should be ventilated 20 times a minute, once every 3 seconds. Newborns should be ventilated 40 times a minute.

54. **c.** Cyanosis and/or an inability to cry are signs that should alert a rescuer to a complete airway obstruction in a conscious infant.

55. **d.** Chest thrusts should be performed on an infant with an airway obstruction, rather than abdominal thrusts.

56. **b.** Perform cycles of five back blows followed by five chest thrusts to relieve an airway obstruction in an infant. If the infant is unconscious, the rescuer should also attempt to ventilate following each set of five chest thrusts. Blind finger sweeps should not be performed on infants or children, as this can push the object back into the airway and cause further obstruction.

57. **b.** Manual removal of foreign bodies obstructing the airway in infants and children should be performed only if the object can be visualized.

58. **d.** The rescuer should keep the infant's head lower than the trunk while performing maneuvers to relieve an obstructed airway. The infant may be straddled over the rescuer's arm to accomplish this.

59. **a.** If a rescuer is alone and finds an infant or child without a pulse and who is not breathing, the patient should be further assessed to see if rescue breathing or CPR is needed. If no one else is available to call EMS, the rescuer should perform CPR for 1 minute, then activate the EMS system. CPR or rescue breathing should be resumed as quickly as possible after the phone call. Since the most common cause of arrest in infants and children is hypoxia, the minute of CPR or rescue breathing may make a critical difference in survival. If another person is present, he or she should immediately activate the EMS system while the rescuer provides medical support.

60. **b.** CPR should not be interrupted for more than a few seconds except in unusual situations. Such situations include moving a patient down stairs or placing an endotracheal tube. CPR must also be interrupted to perform automated external defibrillation.

61. **c.** Fixed and dilated pupils alone are not a reason to stop CPR. CPR may be discontinued if the rescuer is too exhausted to continue, if spontaneous pulses and breathing are restored, or if the patient is pronounced dead by an authorized individual, such as a doctor or a coroner. The responsibility for performing CPR may also be turned over to a higher medical authority, such as a physician or paramedic, but CPR should not be discontinued.

62. **a.** Complications may occur even if compressions are performed correctly by well-trained rescuers. Complications include fractures of the ribs and sternum as well as laceration of the lungs, liver, spleen, and heart and damage to the pleura. Constant practice and skill maintenance can reduce the risk of such complications.

63. **c.** Dentures should normally be left in place when ventilating a patient. Creating a good seal may be difficult if dentures are removed, as they often provide underlying support to the soft tissue of the mouth and face.

64. **c.** If the rescuer notes slight gastric distention during CPR, the airway should be repositioned and ventilation should be delivered less forcefully.

65. **d.** The chance of gastric distention and regurgitation can be reduced by ventilating with less force and speed. On adults, ventilation should be delivered slowly over 1½–2 seconds. Do not continue to force air into the patient after the chest rises.

ADDITIONAL BLS REVIEW

1. Check for <u>unresponsiveness</u> (shake and shout).
2. Access the EMS system.
3. Open <u>airway</u> and check for <u>breathing</u>.
4. Give <u>2 slow breaths</u> if breathing is absent:
   <u>1½ – 2</u> seconds each for adults.
   <u>1 – 1½</u> seconds each for infants and children.
5. Check for <u>breathing</u> and <u>pulse</u>.

Summary of Adult One- and Two-Rescuer CPR

	One–Rescuer	Two–Rescuer
Rate:	80–100 per minute	80–100 per minute
Ratio:	15 compressions/2 breaths	5 compressions/1 breath
Hand Placement:	2 hands: heel of hand 1 or 2 fingers above xyphoid process	2 hands: heel of hand 1 or 2 fingers above xyphoid process
Depth of Compressions:	1½–2 inches	1½–2 inches
Location of Pulse Check:	carotid	carotid
Rescue Breathing:	10–12 times per minute (1 breath every 5–6 seconds)	10–12 times per minute (1 breath every 5–6 seconds)

Summary of Infant and Child CPR

	Infant	Child
Age:	0–1 year	1–8 years
Rate:	>100 per minute	100 per minute
Ratio:	5 compressions/1 breath	5 compressions/1 breath
Hand Placement:	2 or 3 fingers, 1 finger width below line between nipples	Heel of 1 hand: lower third of sternum
Depth of Compressions:	⅓–½ depth of chest approximately ½–1 inch	⅓–½ depth of chest approximately 1–1½ inch
Location of Pulse Check:	brachial	carotid
Rescue Breathing:	20 times per minute (1 breath every 3 seconds)	20 times per minute (1 breath every 3 seconds)

EVALUATION AND SITUATIONAL REVIEW

1. Your unit is summoned to a home for a child who has ingested an unknown quantity of children's aspirin. The patient is a 4-year-old boy. As you question him, you note that he is alert and oriented. You perform an assessment and find no immediately life-threatening problems. He admits to having taken the aspirin, but cannot tell you how much. After telephoning medical direction, you are ordered to administer activated charcoal. The correct dose for this patient is:
   a. 1 mg/kg
   b. 2 g/kg
   c. 12.5–25 grams
   d. 25–50 milligrams

2. Prior to administering the charcoal:
   a. tell the child it is candy
   b. shake the container vigorously
   c. mix the charcoal with water
   d. pour the fluid into a glass

3. Receiving the order to administer activated charcoal is an example of:
   a. up-line medical direction
   b. direct-line medical direction
   c. on-line medical direction
   d. straight-line medical direction

4. The patient is a 28-year-old female in her eighth month of pregnancy. Her family called because she had been complaining of a severe, persistent headache and was vomiting. As you begin your evaluation, you notice that her face and hands are swollen. She is somewhat confused and disoriented, and vital signs reveal a blood pressure of 162/100. Further questioning of the family reveals that the patient experienced sudden weight gain prior to the onset of the other complaints. While caring for this patient, be alert for:
   a. a sudden drop in blood pressure
   b. sudden respiratory arrest
   c. uncontrolled vaginal bleeding
   d. seizures

5. After arriving home from work, a man finds his wife unconscious in bed. The patient is a 28-year-old woman. She responds only to painful stimuli. Her pulse is fast, and she is pale and sweating. The husband tells you she has a history of diabetes. Management of this patient would include:
   a. administering oral glucose
   b. placing the patient on her left side
   c. applying a cervical collar and backboard
   d. placing the patient on oxygen by cannula at 15 lpm

6. It is 2 am. Parents called EMS to evaluate a sick child. Your patient, a 3-year-old, has a cold with only a slight fever. The parents tell you that the child is usually better during the day, but tonight the problem seems worse. As you enter the room, you hear a loud noise that sounds almost like a "seal bark" with each of the child's inspirations. What you hear is:
a. stridor
b. crackles
c. wheezing
d. snoring

7. You attempt to place the child on oxygen, but she does not accept the mask. You try to calm her down, but each time you try to apply the mask she becomes very agitated. You should:
a. leave the child off oxygen to avoid upsetting her
b. restrain the child and place her on oxygen
c. provide oxygen using a blow-by technique
d. place a paper bag over the child's head and place oxygen tubing inside the bag

8. The patient is a 12-year-old boy who sustained a leg injury while playing soccer. Upon examination, you note that the patient's lower leg is painful, swollen, and deformed. After applying a splint and moving the patient to the cot:
a. lower the leg, and apply a heat pack to the injury site
b. elevate the leg, and apply a heat pack to the injury site
c. lower the leg, and apply a cold pack to the injury site
d. elevate the leg, and apply a cold pack to the injury site

9. You are dispatched for a sick child having a seizure. Upon arrival, you find a 2-year-old girl lying on the couch. Her mother tells you she developed a 103-degree temperature relatively quickly. The child has no history of seizures. This seizure was most likely:
a. a febrile seizure
b. due to a head injury
c. a petit mal seizure
d. due to low blood sugar

10. The EMTs should:
a. perform an alcohol rub-down
b. have the parents monitor the child and call back if another seizure occurs
c. transport the child to the hospital for evaluation
d. place the child in a cool bath

11. You have been summoned to the local shopping mall to examine a pregnant female experiencing an "unknown problem." She is pale, her pulse is rapid, and she is complaining of severe, localized abdominal pain. She is in her eighth month of pregnancy. Physical examination reveals steady bleeding from the vagina. The bleeding most likely indicates:
a. a meconium emergency
b. premature labor
c. postpartum hemorrhage
d. a problem with the placenta

12. You are summoned in the morning to check on a patient injured in an auto accident. After arriving at the patient's home, you find that the crash occurred late last evening. The patient is a 16-year-old boy with no history of medical problems. He seems disoriented and occasionally does not respond to verbal stimuli. When he is able to answer your questions, his replies are inappropriate. Family members tell you that the accident occurred just down the road and that the patient was able to walk home. They advise you that, at the time, he seemed to be more concerned that he could not afford car repairs than with any injuries he may have sustained. Your partner examines the car that is now in the driveway and notes a "spiderweb" pattern crack on the driver's side of the windshield. You suspect that his altered mental status is most likely the result of:
a. a head injury
b. a diabetic emergency
c. drinking alcohol
d. seizure activity

13. You are dispatched to a "sick person" at a local restaurant. Upon arrival, you find a female patient reclining in a booth. Friends say that she was talking but suddenly became unresponsive. She is breathing and responds to verbal stimuli, but can only utter sounds. Upon examination you notice that she is unable to move her extremities on the left side, and her mouth tends to droop on the left side. Her vital signs are within normal range. This patient should be transported:
a. in a supine position
b. in a prone position
c. on her left side
d. sitting upright

14. A 54-year-old man is experiencing chest pain and difficulty breathing. The pain started after the patient had walked three flights of stairs to his apartment, which was approximately 10 minutes prior to your being dispatched. The patient states that the pain is mostly on the left side, is radiating down his left arm, and feels like a tremendous pressure. You notice that he is pale and sweating. Part of the care is likely to include:
a. placing the patient on oxygen by cannula at 6 lpm
b. assisting the patient to take nitroglycerin if he has it
c. assisting the patient down the stairs to the stretcher
d. transporting the patient on his back with his legs elevated

15. It is a hot summer day, and your unit is sent to a metal foundry for a "man down." Upon arrival, you find a 22-year-old unresponsive male patient. His pulse is rapid, and he is flushed. His skin is hot and dry to the touch. Management of this patient would include:
a. giving the patient cool water to drink
b. covering the patient with a light blanket to prevent rapid heat loss
c. applying cold packs to the armpits, neck, and groin
d. washing the patient down with rubbing alcohol

16. The local high school has called your unit for a "sick" juvenile in the gymnasium. As you start your evaluation, you find that the patient is conscious but weak and somewhat confused. He is pale and sweating, although his vital signs are normal. His friends tell you that he skipped lunch to play basketball with them. Halfway into the game he became weak, sat down, and soon thereafter started to demonstrate signs of illness. The school nurse arrives with the patient's records and advises you that he does take insulin. You suspect:
a. a drug overdose
b. a head injury
c. a diabetic emergency
d. a heat emergency

17. An important aspect of care for this patient will most likely include:
a. applying cold packs to cool the patient down
b. administering oral glucose
c. checking the patient's locker for illegal drugs
d. placing the patient in the recovery position

18. The patient is a full-term pregnant woman in labor. When you examine the vaginal area, you notice a section of the cord protruding from the vaginal opening. As part of your management, you may need to:
a. tell the patient to push as hard as possible to assist with delivery
b. use two gloved fingers to push the presenting part of the fetus away from the cord
c. pull on the cord
d. tell the patient to cross her legs and not to push

19. The patient should be transported:
a. on her back with the buttocks elevated
b. without using lights and siren
c. on her left side with the head slightly elevated
d. sitting upright

20. You are dispatched to a local retirement home. The patient is a 72-year-old woman who is very independent. She is not pleased that her neighbors have summoned you, but she is obviously having a lot of difficulty breathing. She states that she has been short of breath for about the past 4 hours, but did not want to bother anyone. She has no chest pain. Her pulse rate is 96 and irregular, her blood pressure is 144/82, and her breathing rate is 26 breaths per minute and labored. When you listen to her chest, you note wheezing on both inspiration and expiration. Questioning about medical history reveals that she has a history of emphysema. The correct way to administer oxygen to this patient is by:
    a. nonrebreather mask at 15 lpm
    b. nonrebreather mask at 3 lpm
    c. nasal cannula at 6 lpm
    d. nasal cannula at 3 lpm

21. It is a sunny fall day. The patient is a 9-year-old girl who was outside playing in the leaves with her friends when she developed difficulty breathing. Her parents tell you that she has a history of asthma, but this attack seems much worse than the others. When listening to breath sounds, you hear pronounced wheezing, primarily on expiration. Part of the management of this patient may include:
    a. administering epinephrine
    b. inserting a nasopharyngeal airway
    c. ventilating the patient with a bag-valve-mask
    d. assisting with a prescribed inhaler

22. If this patient's parents were not available to give permission to aid and transport the patient, the EMTs:
    a. could transport but only if a police officer placed the child in protective custody
    b. could aid and transport under the law of implied consent
    c. would have to wait to transport until another blood relative could be contacted
    d. could transport but could not give oxygen or perform any other aid without parental consent

23. Your unit is called to a feed store for a person injured in the storeroom. Your patient is a 15-year-old teenager who was moving inventory when a shelf containing unmarked bags of dry powder fell over. Many of the bags have burst, and your patient is covered with the unknown powder. He is complaining of nausea, abdominal cramps, and moderate difficulty breathing. While performing the examination, you notice that he is sweating and salivating profusely, and his eyes are watery. There is some uncontrolled muscle twitching present. You suspect his problems to be related to:
    a. shock
    b. head injury
    c. chemical poisoning
    d. seizures

24. Early management of the patient would include:
    a. brushing off as much of the powder as possible and washing off the rest
    b. placing the patient in the shock position and conserving body heat
    c. wiping off the powder with a damp rag
    d. wrapping the patient in a plastic sheet

25. It is a typical Friday night at the local gun and knife club, better known as "The East End Bar and Grill." Your patient was on the losing end of a disagreement and received multiple stab wounds to the chest. The knife is still in place. The EMT should:
    a. remove the knife since it may interfere with breathing
    b. apply pressure to the knife to help control bleeding
    c. leave the knife in place and stabilize it with a bulky dressing
    d. place cold packs around the knife blade

26. The other chest wounds should be:
    a. covered only if bleeding is severe
    b. covered with loose, bulky dressings
    c. left uncovered to allow rapid evaluation by hospital personnel
    d. covered with a nonporous dressing

27. Your patient is a 39-year-old man who has been experiencing persistent abdominal pain for the past 12 hours. He has a history of alcoholism but takes no medications. He states that he has been vomiting and that it looks "funny." You notice the vomitus in a trash can, and it resembles coffee grounds. His abdomen is generally tender. Vital signs reveal a slightly rapid pulse and breathing, but blood pressure is normal. You suspect that the patient has:
a. alcohol poisoning
b. internal bleeding
c. appendicitis
d. cardiac compromise

28. The patient states that he is extremely thirsty. You should:
a. avoid giving the patient anything by mouth
b. give the patient water, but less than one cup
c. encourage the patient to drink as much as possible to replenish lost fluids
d. allow the patient to take a drink, but only if the liquid is at room temperature

29. A patient is in active labor. Upon arrival, you follow all the local protocols for handling imminent delivery. Everything seems to be going routinely, but immediately after moving the patient to the litter, her water breaks. You notice that the fluid is thick and resembles pea soup. You become concerned because you are now dealing with a:
a. breech delivery
b. meconium emergency
c. preeclampsia emergency
d. prepartum hemorrhage

30. If the baby delivers before reaching the hospital, your primary action should be to:
a. immediately cut the cord
b. immediately get an APGAR score
c. monitor the mother for seizures
d. aggressively suction the baby's airway

31. You are called to a construction site for a person with a leg injury. You find a 19-year-old man who was struck in the leg by a steel beam. His mid-thigh is painful, swollen, and deformed. Coworkers state that the patient immediately fell to the ground after being struck. The victim tells you that he did not hit his head and denies any neck or back pain. The splint of choice for managing this injury is a:
a. pneumatic splint
b. traction splint
c. soft splint
d. ladder splint

32. A major concern with this type of extremity injury is:
a. there is a high incidence of infection
b. it may become a closed injury
c. serious blood loss
d. amputation below the injury is often indicated

33. The patient is a 72-year-old man who complains of back pain that became increasingly worse since the day before. He tells you that he was weeding his garden and thinks he "just pulled something." His friends called EMS in spite of his objections. He does not want to go to the hospital. You should:
a. explain the possible consequences of his action and allow him to sign a refusal if he still does not want to go
b. restrain the patient and take him to a hospital because he may cause further harm to himself
c. tell him that you are obligated by law to transport him because an ambulance was called
d. request a police officer to arrest the patient, at which time you may transport without his consent

34. You arrive at the scene of a single-car crash and find that the patient has already been removed from the car by bystanders. He is standing and complains of neck and back pain. There is a "spiderweb" crack pattern to the windshield of the vehicle. Your partners have already placed a cervical collar on the patient. The best way to place this patient onto the stretcher is to:
   a. place a backboard on the cot and have the patient sit down on the board
   b. place a short backboard on the patient and then have him lie down on the stretcher
   c. perform an emergency move to place him on the stretcher as quickly as possible
   d. backboard the patient while he is still standing, then move him

35. A 9-year-old boy has just been pulled from the community swimming pool located next door to your station. The lifeguards have been doing CPR for approximately 3 minutes prior to your arrival. Your first actions would include:
   a. attaching the patient to an AED
   b. assessing the adequacy of the CPR being performed
   c. performing abdominal thrusts on the patient
   d. ventilating the patient with a flow-restricted, oxygen-powered device

36. The fire department has removed a man from a burning garage. Upon discovering the fire, the man went through a side door and attempted to open the garage door to remove an antique car. The man is conscious and obviously upset at the firefighters for not allowing him to get the car. As you examine the patient, you notice what appears to be soot or burns around his mouth and nose. The patient is coughing, and his sputum appears to have black particles mixed with it. As he answers some of your questions, he sounds hoarse. He does not want to go to the hospital. You feel he may have:
   a. a diabetic emergency
   b. a closed head injury
   c. an allergic reaction to the smoke
   d. respiratory tract burns

37. Management of this patient would include:
   a. administering oxygen for 15 minutes, and advising him to see his doctor as soon as possible
   b. having him sign a witnessed refusal form, and returning to the station
   c. explaining the complications associated with his problem, and strongly recommending that he go to the hospital to be examined
   d. forcibly restraining him and transporting him to the hospital

38. Your unit is sent to the scene of a person who has fallen down a flight of steps at a college dormitory. The patient is a 20-year-old man who fell approximately ¾ of the way down a long flight of steps. The patient is unconscious and lying on his back at the bottom landing. The patient is assessed, and no external bleeding is noted. Your primary concern is that this patient may:
   a. have a spinal injury
   b. have a history of seizures
   c. be hyperglycemic
   d. be faking unconsciousness

39. You are dispatched to the city park for a person with breathing difficulty. Upon arriving, you encounter a distraught 19-year-old girl who has been stung by a bee. She is complaining of diffuse itching and a tightness in her throat and chest. Physical exam reveals a generalized rash accompanied by hives and a weak, rapid pulse. Wheezing is noted when you listen to the chest. This patient is experiencing:
   a. cardiac compromise
   b. hyperventilation syndrome
   c. an allergic reaction
   d. a diabetic emergency

40. You note that the stinger is still imbedded in the patient's arm. You should:
   a. remove the stinger with a pair of tweezers
   b. leave the stinger in place
   c. cover the stinger with a cold pack
   d. scrape the stinger out using the edge of a card

41. Management of this patient may include assisting with administration of:
a. oral glucose
b. epinephrine
c. activated charcoal
d. nitroglycerine

42. Before assisting with this particular medication, it is important to check:
a. the medication's date of manufacture
b. to be sure that the patient is not allergic to the medication
c. the expiration date of the medication
d. the name of the doctor who prescribed the medication

43. Your patient is an 82-year-old woman with severe difficulty breathing. As you enter the house, you hear gurgling breathing from the back bedroom. She is sitting upright in bed and coughing up frothy sputum. When you listen to her chest, you hear wet breath sounds. She has difficulty speaking, but denies any pain. You notice her neck veins are distended, and examination of her ankles and feet reveal marked swelling. This patient should be transported:
a. supine and on high-flow oxygen
b. sitting upright and on high-flow oxygen
c. laying flat and on oxygen via cannula
d. in a position of comfort and on low-flow oxygen

44. You are called to the scene of a chain saw accident. A 31-year-old man was working in a tree when the saw hit his thigh. His coworkers helped him out of the tree, but he is still bleeding profusely. The first attempts to control bleeding should be performed using:
a. arterial pressure points
b. a tourniquet
c. venous pressure points
d. direct pressure over the wound

45. It is the first cold day of winter. Along with the fire department, you respond to a call for a furnace explosion. The owner was asleep when he heard a loud bang in the basement and awoke to find smoke billowing from the heat registers. He was not burned or injured, but tells you he has a severe headache, nausea, and "feels real bad." He denies having felt that way before he went to bed. He was the sole occupant of the house. You suspect that the patient is suffering from:
a. the flu
b. a head injury
c. inhalation poisoning
d. a nervous disorder

46. Initial management would include:
a. administering high-flow oxygen by nonrebreather mask
b. applying a cervical collar
c. placing the patient in Trendelenburg position
d. cooling the patient

47. A patient was recently released from the hospital after undergoing abdominal surgery. The patient had a coughing spell that caused the stitches to rupture. Upon arrival, you find part of the man's intestines protruding from the open incision. Management would include:
a. replacing the organs in the abdominal cavity
b. covering the organs with a moist, sterile dressing
c. applying direct pressure on the organs to prevent internal bleeding
d. covering the organs with a dry, sterile dressing

48. The patient should be transported:
a. on his left side with the knees and hips flexed
b. sitting up with his knees straight
c. on his back with the knees and hips flexed
d. on his right side with the knees and hips straight

49. It's another Friday night at the local high school football game. As usual, your team is losing. You and your partner are standing by at the game trying to make the best of the last 10 minutes before returning to the station when spectators nearby start yelling that someone has "passed out." It takes you only about a minute to reach a 58-year-old man who is in cardiac arrest. Your first action is to:
a. attach the patient to an AED
b. begin two-rescuer CPR
c. place the patient on oxygen
d. insert an oral airway

50. You are dispatched to a possible behavioral emergency. When you enter the house, police are already on the scene arguing with a 43-year-old man. You notice that the inside of the house has been demolished. The patient tells you that foreign agents are trying to kill him by letting tarantulas loose in the house. From time to time, the patient claims to see one going under a piece of overturned furniture. He also tells you that the agents operate out of the local hospital and that he is not going to be taken alive. Discussion with the patient's family reveals that he has a long history of behavioral problems and that he has not been taking his prescribed medication. He also has a history of violence. You should:
a. offer to help the patient kill all the tarantulas if he goes with you to the hospital
b. tell him you are just taking him to see his family doctor
c. join the police in arguing with him about going to the hospital
d. consider restraining the patient

51. You arrive at a scene involving a female patient experiencing chest pain. The patient is complaining of substernal chest pain radiating to the left arm. She was cleaning the house when the pain started. She is on an unknown medication for high blood pressure but takes no other prescribed drug. Her vital signs are normal, and she complains of only minimal shortness of breath. Her husband has a history of heart problems, and she advises you that she has access to his nitroglycerin. Your actions should include:
a. contacting medical direction for permission to assist the patient with taking the nitroglycerine
b. placing the patient on high-flow oxygen by nonrebreather mask
c. placing the patient on an AED
d. contacting the patient's family doctor for further instructions

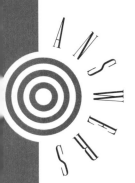

17 EVALUATION

AND SITUATIONAL REVIEW

1. **c.** The correct dose is 12.5–25 grams, or 1g/kg.

2. **b.** Prior to administering the charcoal, shake the container vigorously. Do not lie to the child by saying it is candy. Also, do not put the charcoal in a glass because if the child sees the slurry, he may not be willing to drink it.

3. **c.** The order received over the telephone was an example of on-line medical direction.

4. **d.** The EMT should be alert for seizures.

5. **b.** The patient should be placed on her left side to facilitate drainage of secretions from the mouth. Because she is unresponsive, she should not be given oral glucose. Oxygen is indicated, but by nonrebreather mask at 15 lpm.

6. **a.** The sound is stridor, and it indicates an upper–airway problem.

7. **c.** Because the child will not tolerate the oxygen mask, administer oxygen using a blow-by technique to enrich the air in the immediate vicinity of the child's mouth and nose.

8. **d.** After applying a splint, elevate the leg and apply cold packs to the area. This will help reduce swelling.

9. **a.** The child has most likely suffered a febrile seizure.

10. **c.** The child should be taken to a hospital for evaluation. Although a febrile seizure is suspected, other causes should be ruled out by a doctor.

11. **d.** Vaginal bleeding that occurs during late pregnancy is usually associated with a problem with the placenta.

12. **a.** The patient's altered mental status is most likely the result of a head injury that occurred in the auto crash. The "spiderweb" pattern on the windshield indicates that the patient's head has struck the windshield.

13. **c.** Because the patient may be unable to protect her airway, she should be transported on the left side.

14. **b.** If the patient has a prescription for nitroglycerin, you will probably be instructed to assist the patient in taking the medication.

15. c. This patient is experiencing a serious medical problem. Because rapid cooling is needed, cold packs should be applied to the armpits, neck, and groin area.

16. c. The patient is most likely experiencing a diabetic emergency.

17. b. Administration of oral glucose will probably be ordered.

18. b. Management of a prolapsed cord may include inserting two gloved fingers into the vagina to push the presenting part of the fetus away from the cord, thereby taking pressure off the cord.

19. a. Transport the patient on her back with the buttocks elevated, which will allow gravity to assist in taking some pressure off the cord. Because this is a true emergency situation, transport should be done with lights and sirens unless contraindicated by local protocols.

20. a. This patient needs a lot of oxygen. Use a nonrebreather mask at 15 lpm.

21. d. Since this patient has a history of asthma, she may have a prescribed inhaler. If so, medical direction will probably order you to assist her in using it.

22. b. Even if the parents are not present, care and transport can proceed under the law of implied consent. A police officer does not have to be present.

23. c. The patient's problems are probably related to some sort of chemical poisoning.

24. a. Because the poison is entering the skin through absorption, it must be removed. Brush off as much of the chemical as possible, then wash off any remaining chemical with copious amounts of water. The patient's clothing should be removed. Wrapping the patient in a plastic sheet would keep the poison near the patient and allow continued absorption.

25. c. The knife should be left in place and stabilized with a bulky dressing.

26. d. The other chest wounds should be covered with nonporous dressings.

27. b. This patient is displaying signs of internal bleeding.

28. a. Although the patient is extremely thirsty, give no fluids by mouth because the patient may need to go into surgery. Even if he does not, the fluids may worsen the nausea.

29. b. Discharge of amniotic fluid that resembles thick, green pea soup indicates a meconium emergency.

30. d. Aggressive suctioning is a must. Particular attention to the baby's airway is crucial to keep the meconium from entering the lungs.

31. b. This type of musculoskeletal injury is best managed with a traction splint. A traction splint should not be used, however, if the injury is close to the knee or hip; if a partial amputation or avulsion with bone separation is present; or if the ankle, lower leg, knee, or pelvis is also injured.

32. c. A femur injury of this type can result in severe blood loss. The injury is a closed injury, but mismanagement may turn it into an open injury.

33. a. Rational adult patients have the right to refuse any or all care. Thorough documentation is important whenever a patient refuses transport.

34. d. This patient should be backboarded while still standing. Although he was moving around at the scene, a spinal injury may still be present.

35. b. Upon arrival, assess the adequacy of the CPR being performed. This patient is too young for the AED or flow-restricted, oxygen-powered ventilation. Abdominal thrusts are not indicated in the initial management of all drowning patients.

36. d. The patient probably has respiratory tract burns. Signs include a history of being in an enclosed fire area, soot or burns around the mouth and nose, coughing accompanied by black particles in the sputum, and hoarseness.

37. c. Explain the potential complications and strongly recommend that the patient go to the hospital. Also, keep the patient on high-flow oxygen for as long as possible.

38. a. The patient's presentation strongly suggests a spinal injury.

39. c. The patient is experiencing an allergic reaction. Clues include a bee sting, diffuse itching, tightness in the throat and chest, rash and hives, a rapid pulse, and wheezing.

40. d. Scrape the stinger out using the edge of a card or something similar. Using tweezers may force more poison into the wound. Do not leave the stinger in place, as muscles around the poison sac may continue to constrict, thereby forcing more poison into the patient.

41. b. Management of this patient may include administering epinephrine if it has been prescribed for the patient.

42. c. Check the expiration date of the epinephrine before administering it. There are no contraindications to using epinephrine in a life-threatening situation.

43. b. The patient has fluid in her lungs and should be transported sitting upright to allow gravity to keep the upper lungs as clear as possible. She also needs high-flow oxygen.

44. d. Attempts at controlling bleeding should initially be done by applying direct pressure to the wound area.

45. c. The patient is most likely suffering from inhalation poisoning.

46. a. The patient should immediately be given 15 lpm of oxygen by nonrebreather mask.

47. b. Management of an evisceration includes covering the organs with a moist, sterile dressing.

48. c. The patient should be transported on his back with the hips and knees flexed.

49. **a.** Early defibrillation is the key in managing this patient. If an AED is readily available, defibrillation takes priority over ensuring an adequate airway and performing CPR. If two EMTs are present, one can start one-rescuer CPR while the other connects the AED.

50. **d.** Due to the violent nature of this patient's behavior, restraint is probably needed to protect the patient as well as the rescuers. Do not argue with or lie to the patient, and do not go along with his hallucinations.

51. **b.** The patient should be placed on high-flow oxygen. Because she does not have her own prescription for nitroglycerine, she should not be assisted in taking it.

CHAPTER 18

100 QUESTION PRACTICE TEST

1. You are caring for a patient with an obvious head injury due to trauma. During your assessment, you note that the patient has low blood pressure and a rapid pulse. You should:
   a. position the patient on the right side with the head lower than the feet
   b. suspect other injuries or bleeding
   c. place the patient in a sitting position
   d. suspect a diabetic emergency

2. A patient with a minor injury, such as an ankle injury, should receive:
   a. an initial assessment followed by a focused history and physical exam
   b. an initial assessment only
   c. a detailed assessment only
   d. a focused history and physical exam followed by a detailed assessment

3. Perform an emergency move when:
   a. the patient's condition may deteriorate
   b. there are not enough EMTs to properly move the patient
   c. there is an immediate threat to the life of the patient
   d. maximum control of the spine is needed

4. Bleeding that spurts with each heartbeat and is bright red in color is characteristic of:
   a. arterial bleeding
   b. primary bleeding
   c. venous bleeding
   d. consecutive bleeding

5. A patient with a broken-down car was stranded in freezing weather. To manage the late (or deep) cold–related injuries:
   a. apply heat to the injured areas
   b. break any blisters that may have formed
   c. rub or massage the affected areas
   d. cover the areas with dry dressings

6. During your examination of a 4-year-old child experiencing difficulty breathing, you note wheezing on expiration. You suspect that this is caused by:
   a. throat inflammation
   b. upper airway obstruction
   c. lower airway disease
   d. dilated bronchioles

7. A patient is semiconscious and having difficulty maintaining an airway; however, she still has a gag reflex. The airway you would consider using is the:
   a. oropharyngeal airway
   b. nasopharyngeal airway
   c. PTL airway
   d. endotracheal airway

8. Contraindication refers to:
   a. the way a medication affects the body
   b. a side effect of a medication
   c. a medication that acts in the opposite way when administered with a different drug
   d. a situation in which a medication should not be administered because it may cause harm

9. Following delivery of a healthy infant, you prepare to cut the umbilical cord. The first clamp should be placed about:
   a. 5 inches from the mother
   b. 5 inches from the baby
   c. 10 inches from the mother
   d. 10 inches from the baby

10. After taking appropriate body substance isolation precautions, the first step in controlling bleeding is:
    a. placing the patient in the shock position
    b. application of direct pressure
    c. digital pressure on an artery
    d. cold application

11. When performing two-rescuer adult CPR, compressions are delivered at a rate of:
    a. 40–60 per minute
    b. 60–80 per minute
    c. 80–100 per minute
    d. at least 120 per minute

12. Your patient has a history of violent behavior and is extremely agitated. The best course of management is to:
    a. approach the patient alone to gain his confidence
    b. surprise the patient and overpower him
    c. threaten the patient with physical harm if he becomes violent
    d. approach the patient only with backup assistance

13. A pedestrian has been struck by a car and is in shock. As part of the care rendered:
    a. control bleeding after ensuring an adequate airway and that the patient is breathing
    b. place the patient on oxygen after splinting fractures
    c. apply heating pads or hot water bottles to keep the patient warm
    d. check vital signs every 15 minutes

14. The method used to determine the correct size of oral airway to insert is to measure from the:
    a. patient's Adam's apple to the corner of the mouth
    b. patient's earlobe to the corner of the mouth
    c. angle of the patient's jaw to the Adam's apple
    d. angle of the patient's jaw to the clavicle

15. An EMT may insert fingers into a pregnant patient's vagina:
    a. to support the baby's head during delivery
    b. to assist the delivery of the shoulders
    c. only in the case of a breech delivery or prolapsed cord
    d. to check the baby's pulse in the event of a meconium emergency

16. Ventilate an adult patient who is not breathing but has a pulse at a rate of:
    a. 6–10 times a minute, once every 6–10 seconds
    b. 10–12 times a minute, once every 5–6 seconds
    c. 12–15 times a minute, once every 4–5 seconds
    d. 15–20 times a minute, once every 3–4 seconds

17. A patient with vomitus resembling coffee grounds should be suspected of having:
    a. appendicitis
    b. internal bleeding
    c. diverticulitis
    d. gallbladder problems

18. A male patient is hypothermic but is alert and responding appropriately. Care for the patient would include:
    a. having him walk vigorously
    b. massaging his arms and legs to stimulate circulation
    c. rewarming him by applying heat packs to the neck, armpit, and groin area
    d. giving him hot coffee or alcohol to drink

19. You and your partners have returned from a run involving a SIDS patient. If a Critical Incident Stress Management team is needed, it should be requested:
    a. 1–2 weeks from the incident
    b. within a month of the incident
    c. no later than 24 hours after the incident
    d. Within 24–72 hours after the incident

20. When a patient with a skeletal injury and no distal pulses is encountered:
    a. realign the injury using gentle traction
    b. never straighten the injury
    c. realign the injury while pushing on the limb
    d. splint the injury with a traction splint

21. When using the mnemonic S-A-M-P-L-E, the letter "E" refers to:
    a. how long it took "EMS" to arrive
    b. whether the problem is a true "emergency"
    c. the "events" leading up to the injury or illness
    d. whether the patient was "extricated"

22. A nasal cannula may be used when:
    a. the patient complains of a dry mouth
    b. the patient does not tolerate a nonrebreather mask
    c. pressure in the oxygen tank is too low to use a mask
    d. the patient is breathing primarily through the nose

23. To perform chest compressions on an infant, use:
    a. two fingers placed on the upper sternum
    b. the heel of one hand placed on the middle of the sternum
    c. two fingers placed one finger width below the nipple line
    d. both thumbs placed on the upper sternum

24. When performing an assessment of a child, the most important thing is the:
    a. patient's pulse rate
    b. parent's reaction
    c. patient's blood pressure
    d. EMT's general impression of the patient's well-being

25. Proper lifting should be performed using the:
    a. arms while keeping the feet as far apart as possible
    b. legs while keeping the feet shoulder-width apart
    c. waist while keeping the feet together
    d. back while keeping the feet shoulder-width apart

26. When a nonrebreather mask is used, the proper oxygen flow rate is:
    a. 3 lpm if there is a history of difficulty breathing
    b. 6 lpm if the patient does not tolerate high flow
    c. 9 lpm if the patient complains of a dry mouth and nose
    d. 15 lpm in all cases

27. A patient has just depressed her handheld inhaler and begins to inhale deeply. Immediately after the medication has been delivered, instruct the patient to:
    a. hold her breath
    b. exhale forcefully
    c. cough vigorously
    d. swallow

28. A wound characterized by irregular, jagged edges is:
    a. an avulsion
    b. a laceration
    c. an amputation
    d. an abrasion

29. Wear protective eyewear:
    a. whenever a patient with an infectious disease is encountered
    b. if the patient has TB
    c. if the EMT was recently ill
    d. in situations where blood may splatter

30. During the assessment, you decide that you are dealing with a priority patient. Your action would be to:
    a. call an ALS unit for assistance and wait at the scene for its arrival
    b. immediately transport to the hospital of the patient's choice
    c. call medical control and request further instructions for on-scene management
    d. expedite transport to an appropriate medical facility

31. An 18-year-old man has been involved in a fight and has a knife protruding from the abdomen. Management of the impaled object would include:
    a. stabilizing it with a bulky dressing
    b. applying pressure to it for bleeding control
    c. removing it immediately
    d. packing ice around it

32. A 16-year-old female experienced a seizure while sitting on the couch. She is still unresponsive. Because your assessment reveals no reasons to suspect spinal injury, the position of choice to transport this patient is:
    a. prone
    b. supine
    c. in the recovery position
    d. in the shock position

33. Restlessness and anxiety, a rapid pulse, cool, clammy skin, and a drop in blood pressure are signs of:
    a. hyperglycemia
    b. a brain injury
    c. an impending seizure
    d. hypoperfusion

34. Most accidents involving emergency vehicles occur:
    a. due to skids
    b. at intersections
    c. during U-turns
    d. en route to the hospital

35. For CPR on infants or children, the ratio of compressions to ventilations is:
    a. 5:1 for infants and 15:2 for children
    b. 15:2 regardless of the number of rescuers
    c. 5:1 regardless of the number of rescuers
    d. 15:2 for one-rescuer CPR

36. Generally, joint injuries should be:
    a. realigned prior to splinting
    b. stabilized with a traction splint
    c. splinted in the position found
    d. transported without splinting to reduce aggravation

37. Assistance may be rendered to an unconscious patient under the law of:
    a. implied consent
    b. actual consent
    c. informed consent
    d. minor's consent

38. A 25-year-old construction worker has been struck in the mid-thigh by a steel beam. He is complaining of severe pain in the thigh area. The splint of choice for this injury is:
    a. a soft splint
    b. a pneumatic splint
    c. a traction splint
    d. an air splint

39. When using a tourniquet, remember that it should be:
    a. placed below a knee or elbow if a foot or hand is bleeding severely
    b. used whenever direct pressure alone does not control bleeding
    c. used whenever an amputation is encountered
    d. used only as a last resort

40. The first thing that should be done for a burn patient is to:
    a. stop the burning process
    b. apply sterile burn sheets
    c. estimate the percentage of burns
    d. assess breathing and circulation

41. After determining that an adult patient is not breathing, deliver:
    a. four quick breaths
    b. two slow breaths if alone, four quick breaths if a partner is present
    c. one full breath 1 to 1½ seconds in duration
    d. two full breaths 1½ to 2 seconds in duration

42. When a patient has bruising around the eyes or behind the ears, suspect:
    a. a skull injury
    b. high blood pressure
    c. a history of violence
    d. a seizure disorder

43. Systolic pressure is:
    a. the difference between the resting pressure and pumping pressure
    b. the pressure exerted against the walls of the arteries during ventricular contraction
    c. the pressure exerted against the walls of the arteries when the left ventricle is at rest
    d. double the diastolic pressure

44. Your patient was the victim of an assault and has been struck a number of times in the head with a baseball bat. He is bleeding from the nose and ears. During the exam, be alert for:
    a. synovial fluid
    b. saline fluid
    c. cerebrospinal fluid
    d. aqueous fluid

45. If a patient does not have a suspected spinal injury, the preferred method of opening the airway is the:
    a. head tilt/chin lift
    b. modified jaw thrust
    c. Heimlich maneuver
    d. head tilt/neck lift

46. Bleeding from an open or depressed skull injury is best controlled by:
    a. applying firm pressure to the wound
    b. applying digital pressure to both carotid arteries
    c. packing the wound with gauze
    d. using a loose, bulky dressing

47. You have been ordered to assist a patient with administering medication. Before doing so:
    a. be sure that it was prescribed by a local doctor
    b. check the expiration date
    c. note what pharmacy dispensed the prescription
    d. be sure the prescription belongs to someone in the patient's family

48. The assessment of a responsive patient:
    a. can usually wait until the patient is moved to the ambulance
    b. emphasizes the patient's vital signs
    c. is normally based on the patient's primary complaint
    d. is not as critical if there is no history of medical problems

49. Patients experiencing cardiac problems most commonly describe the pain as:
    a. pressure or a crushing feeling
    b. made worse by by inhaling deeply
    c. a sharp, stabbing, knife-like pain
    d. cramping and intermittent

50. The primary goal of a detailed assessment is to:
    a. check for signs of physical abuse or drug use
    b. help the EMT diagnose the patient's problem
    c. confirm that a medical problem exists
    d. find less serious injuries or medical problems that may be hidden

51. A patient with an altered mental status is encountered. After assuring scene safety, the first priority in managing this patient is to:
a. administer sugar
b. assure an adequate airway
c. perform a focused exam
d. assess baseline vitals

52. You are preparing a male patient for transport. He has an evisceration but no accompanying spinal or leg injuries. The preferred position for this patient is on his:
a. stomach with the hips and knees straight
b. back with the hips and knees flexed
c. left side
d. right side

53. A patient is experiencing chest pain and has possession of his own nitroglycerin. Before taking the medication, the patient's blood pressure should be:
a. no more than 70 diastolic
b. at least 90 diastolic
c. greater than 100 systolic
d. no more than 130 systolic

54. The airway of a patient with a suspected neck injury should be opened using the:
a. modified jaw thrust
b. head tilt/chin lift
c. head tilt/neck lift
d. Heimlich maneuver

55. A 3-year-old child is having obvious difficulty breathing and is noted to be cyanotic. He does not tolerate an oxygen mask. Your best option is to:
a. restrain the child and force him to wear the mask
b. wait for the child to become unconscious, then administer oxygen
c. administer oxygen using a blow-by technique
d. ventilate the patient with a flow-restricted, oxygen-powered ventilation device

56. You are caring for a conscious patient with a history of diabetes and an altered mental status. Management of this patient is likely to include:
a. applying a cervical collar
b. assisting with use of a prescribed inhaler
c. oxygen by nonrebreather mask at 6 lpm
d. administering oral glucose

57. A patient has fallen from a roof and presents with multiple musculoskeletal injuries and hypoperfusion. You would:
a. splint all injuries prior to moving the patient to prevent further blood loss
b. perform full-body immobilization with a backboard and transport immediately
c. splint only open musculoskeletal injuries prior to moving the patient
d. move the patient to the ambulance cot in whatever way necessary and transport rapidly

58. During transport, patients without spinal injuries experiencing difficulty breathing should be placed:
a. flat on the back
b. on the left side
c. in a position of comfort
d. in the Trendelenburg position

59. All injured and unconscious patients should be suspected of having:
a. spinal injury
b. high blood sugar
c. heart problems
d. taken an overdose

60. To perform chest compressions on a child, use:
a. the heel of one hand placed on the upper half of the sternum
b. two hands placed on the middle of the sternum
c. three fingers below the nipple line
d. the heel of one hand placed on the lower third of the sternum

61. Early management of an open chest injury includes:
a. covering the wound with a loose, bulky dressing
b. sealing the wound with a nonporous dressing
c. supporting the injured area with sandbags
d. placing the patient on a backboard

62. A patient is found unconscious in a garage with a car still running, and is thus a victim of poison gas inhalation. After assuring personal safety and reaching the patient, the EMT's first step in caring for this patient is to:
a. place a cervical collar on the patient
b. remove the patient from the toxic environment
c. determine the type of gas involved
d. open the airway and assess breathing

63. A restrained patient starts spitting at the EMTs during transportation. This can be managed by:
a. using surgical tape to secure the patient's mouth shut
b. placing a pillow over the patient's face
c. covering the patient's mouth with a surgical mask
d. using a cravat to tie the patient's jaw shut

64. Upon reaching a cardiac arrest victim, automated external defibrillation should be performed (if an AED is available):
a. after CPR has been performed for 1 minute
b. unless bystander CPR is being performed
c. after an oral airway is inserted
d. immediately

65. A patient has a severe laceration to the forearm, and direct pressure does not adequately control the bleeding. The pressure point of choice for this patient is the:
a. temporal artery
b. popliteal artery
c. brachial artery
d. tibial artery

66. Suspicions of child abuse should be:
a. reported to the child's parents
b. privately reported to the appropriate authorities
c. reported to the dispatcher
d. anonymously reported by letter to child welfare authorities

67. Proper insertion of an oral airway in an adult may entail inserting the airway:
a. upside-down and then rotating it 180 degrees
b. by pushing the tip along the tongue
c. until the flange lies immediately behind the teeth
d. so the flange lies 1 inch beyond the lips

68. After completing an initial assessment on an unresponsive medical patient, perform:
a. an assessment beginning with the chest to evaluate the lungs and heart
b. a thorough, detailed physical exam
c. a rapid head-to-toe assessment similar to the rapid trauma assessment
d. an abbreviated focused history

69. When suctioning a newborn:
a. wait until delivery is complete to perform suctioning
b. squeeze the bulb syringe before inserting it
c. insert the tip 2–3 inches into the mouth and each nostril
d. lubricate the bulb syringe with petroleum jelly

70. When using O-P-Q-R-S-T to assess a patient, "Provocation" refers to:
a. what time the pain started
b. what makes the pain feel better or worse
c. whether the patient has a violent history or easily loses his temper
d. whether the patient has a previous injury or medical condition

71. An important early step in caring for a patient with skin that is hot to the touch is to:
   a. conserve body heat to avoid rebound hypothermia
   b. wipe down the patient with rubbing alcohol
   c. keep the skin dry
   d. apply cold packs to the neck, groin, and armpits

72. You encounter a patient who is complaining of respiratory distress, a tight feeling in the throat, and itching. The exam reveals wheezing in the lungs and hives on the patient's arms. This patient is probably experiencing:
   a. cardiac problems
   b. a drug overdose
   c. an allergic reaction
   d. a diabetic emergency

73. When transporting a pregnant woman with a spinal injury on a backboard, the backboard should:
   a. be tilted to the right
   b. be tilted to the left
   c. allow for elevation of the head
   d. be completely flat

74. The EMT should evaluate motor, sensory, and circulatory status of an injured extremity:
   a. before and after splinting
   b. only if there is numbness or loss of sensation below the injury site
   c. only if a deformity is present
   d. only before splinting

75. CPR is being performed on a child who is not breathing. Concerning the use of an oral airway in a child, remember:
   a. to insert the airway upside-down and rotate it once after it is in the proper position
   b. that medical control must order its use
   c. to insert the airway right-side–up without using the rotating maneuver that would be used for placement in an adult
   d. that oral airways should not be used

76. Reddening, blister formation, and intense pain is characteristic of a:
   a. superficial burn
   b. partial-thickness burn
   c. medium-thickness burn
   d. full-thickness burn

77. A patient has been exposed to toxic gas. A major concern in dealing with this patient is that when a poison has been inhaled:
   a. activated charcoal should be administered within an hour
   b. it takes longer to enter the blood stream
   c. oxygen should not be administered to the patient
   d. it may also damage the lining of the patient's airway

78. The ratio of chest compressions to ventilations in one-rescuer adult CPR is:
   a. 5:2
   b. 15:2
   c. 5:1
   d. 15:1

79. A 22-year-old male has been stabbed and presents with an evisceration. Management would include:
   a. applying a moist, sterile dressing to the area and covering it with an occlusive dressing
   b. replacing the organs in the abdominal cavity
   c. applying direct pressure to the organs and wound to control bleeding
   d. applying the PASG and inflating all three compartments

80. A patient's eyes that have been burned by chemicals should be irrigated:
   a. with a neutralizing solution
   b. for no longer than 15 minutes
   c. until the patient reaches the hospital
   d. only at the scene of the incident

81. A contraindication for giving oral glucose is:
   a. a blood pressure below 120 systolic
   b. a history of diabetes
   c. if the patient takes insulin
   d. if the patient is unable to swallow

82. A patient has been poisoned by contact with a powdered chemical. One aspect of management includes:
   a. leaving the chemical in place so the hospital can identify it
   b. brushing off any chemical
   c. removing the chemical with a wet towel
   d. wrapping the patient in a blanket to prevent spread of the chemical

83. You and your partner have just delivered a baby. The umbilical cord should be clamped and cut:
   a. after pulsations in the cord cease
   b. before the infant starts breathing
   c. after delivery of the placenta
   d. 10–15 minutes after delivery

84. A 32-year-old male has had a finger cut off in an industrial accident. The proper way to package the finger for transportation to the hospital is to:
   a. pack the finger in ice
   b. immerse the finger in sterile water
   c. wrap the finger in a sterile dressing and keep it cool
   d. wrap the finger in a wet, sterile dressing and keep it warm

85. In essence, the ongoing assessment repeats all the components of the:
   a. detailed physical exam
   b. rapid trauma assessment
   c. S-A-M-P-L-E history
   d. initial assessment

86. A dire emergency exists if a patient has:
   a. moist, pale, normal temperature skin
   b. dry or moist, hot temperature skin
   c. moist, pale, cool temperature skin
   d. moist, pink, normal temperature skin

87. The normal breathing rate for an adult is:
   a. 5–10 breaths per minute
   b. 8–16 breaths per minute
   c. 12–20 breaths per minute
   d. 16–28 breaths per minute

88. The EMT should consider delivery imminent when:
   a. contractions are less than 2 minutes apart
   b. it is the mother's first pregnancy and contractions are 5 minutes apart
   c. contractions last longer than 20 seconds
   d. the patient is experiencing lower abdominal pain with no back pain

89. You are preparing to transport a child with a gastrostomy tube. The two positions in which the patient may be transported are:
   a. lying on the back, or lying on the left side with the head lower than the trunk
   b. in a position of comfort, or prone with the head lower than the trunk
   c. sitting, or lying on the right side with the head elevated
   d. supine, or prone with the head elevated

90. A condition in which the body is unable to utilize glucose normally is:
   a. asthma
   b. diabetes
   c. epistaxis
   d. appendicitis

91. Ideally, the detailed physical examination should be performed:
   a. prior to leaving for the hospital
   b. after ALS personnel arrive
   c. before moving the patient
   d. en route to the hospital

92. You and your partner are sent to evaluate a female patient experiencing a behavioral emergency. The patient may exhibit violent behavior if you find her:
a. sitting on the edge of a seat
b. laying on a bed or couch
c. using monotone speech
d. exhibiting open hands

93. Medical command advises you to administer activated charcoal to an adult patient. The usual dose is:
a. 12.5–25 grams
b. 25–50 grams
c. 50–75 grams
d. 75–100 grams

94. To relieve an airway obstruction in an infant, perform cycles of:
a. Six to ten abdominal thrusts
b. Five back blows followed by five abdominal thrusts
c. Six to ten chest thrusts followed by a finger sweep
d. Five back blows followed by five chest thrusts

95. A burn to the entire leg of an adult would comprise:
a. 6% of body surface area
b. 12% of body surface area
c. 18% of body surface area
d. 24% of body surface area

96. An indication for the use of the PASG would be hypotension and:
a. an unstable pelvic injury
b. an open chest wound
c. abdominal pain
d. arterial bleeding

97. When caring for a sick or injured child:
a. never allow parents to be present
b. allow parents to be present only if absolutely necessary
c. make judicious use of the parents to assist
d. allow only one parent to be present at any time

98. Cardiac muscle differs from other muscles because it:
a. is a voluntary type of muscle
b. can tolerate interruption of blood supply for long periods of time
c. is only found in the heart and lungs
d. has the ability to contract on its own

99. You and your partner are the first to arrive at the scene of an overturned truck carrying a hazardous material. Identification of the material can best be made by:
a. calling the EPA
b. referencing the number on the placard
c. smelling or feeling the substance
d. obtaining a sample and sending it to a laboratory

100. The operation of log-rolling a patient is usually directed by:
a. the EMT at the patient's waist
b. the EMT at the patient's shoulders
c. the EMT controlling the patient's head and neck
d. the senior EMT on the crew

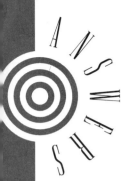

18 100 QUESTION

PRACTICE TEST

NOTE: More information on specific questions may be found by referencing the corresponding chapter and question number.

	ANSWER	CHAPTER	QUESTION
1.	b.	13	23
2.	a.	4	51
3.	c.	15	32
4.	a.	10	14
5.	d.	7	44
6.	c.	14	22
7.	b.	3	23
8.	d.	5	4
9.	d.	9	21
10.	b.	10	16
11.	c.	16	28

	ANSWER	CHAPTER	QUESTION
12.	d.	8	18
13.	a.	10	8
14.	b.	3	25
15.	c.	9	13
16.	b.	16	11
17.	b.	10	31
18.	c.	7	37
19.	d.	15	72
20.	a.	12	11
21.	c.	2	43
22.	b.	3	16
23.	c.	16	50

	ANSWER	CHAPTER	QUESTION		ANSWER	CHAPTER	QUESTION
24.	d.	2	2	42.	a.	13	22
25.	b.	15	22 & 24	43.	b.	2	33
26.	d.	3	14	44.	c.	13	26
27.	a.	5	20	45.	a.	16	7
28.	b.	11	4	46.	d.	13	27
29.	d.	15	61	47.	b.	5	2
30.	d.	4	19	48.	c.	4	41
31.	a.	11	14	49.	a.	5	23
32.	c.	6	24	50.	d.	4	50
33.	d.	10	6	51.	b.	6	2
34.	b.	15	12	52.	b.	11	21
35.	c.	16	52	53.	c.	5	34
36.	c.	12	13	54.	a.	16	8
37.	a.	15	3	55.	c.	3	22
38.	c.	12	19	56.	d.	6	10
39.	d.	10	22	57.	b.	12	5
40.	a.	11	55	58.	c.	5	15
41.	d.	16	10	59.	a.	13	1

	ANSWER	CHAPTER	QUESTION		ANSWER	CHAPTER	QUESTION
60.	d.	16	42	78.	b.	16	20
61.	b.	11	16	79.	a.	11	20
62.	b.	7	11	80.	c.	11	63
63.	c.	8	24	81.	d.	6	12
64.	d.	5	37	82.	b.	7	17
65.	c.	10	19	83.	a.	9	20
66.	b.	14	43	84.	c.	11	24
67.	a.	3	26	85.	d.	4	60
68.	c.	4	40	86.	b.	7	52
69.	b.	9	15	87.	c.	2	7
70.	b.	4	43	88.	a.	9	9
71.	d.	7	54	89.	c.	14	47
72.	c.	6	26	90.	b.	6	4
73.	b.	9	42	91.	d.	4	57
74.	a.	12	6	92.	a.	8	14
75.	c.	14	13	93.	b.	7	24
76.	b.	11	38	94.	d.	16	56
77.	d.	7	10	95.	c.	11	39

	ANSWER	CHAPTER	QUESTION			ANSWER	CHAPTER	QUESTION
96.	**a.**	12	26		99.	**b.**	15	75
97.	**c.**	14	4		100.	**c.**	13	9
98.	**d.**	1	22					